LEANING on GOD'S HEART

Other books by this author:

No More Broken Places
Staying Vertical
Write It on Your Heart

To order, **call 1–800–765–6955.**

Visit us at www.reviewandherald.com
for information on other Review and Herald® products.

When Nothing Is Left,
You Still Have
God

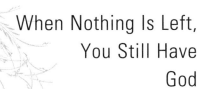

LEANING
on GOD'S
HEART

CAROLYN SUTTON

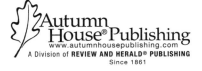

Autumn House® Publishing
www.autumnhousepublishing.com
A Division of **REVIEW AND HERALD® PUBLISHING**
Since 1861

Published by Autumn House® Publishing, a division of Review and Herald® Publishing,
Hagerstown, MD 21741-1119

Autumn House® titles may be purchased in bulk for educational, business, fund-raising, or
sales promotional use. For information, please e-mail SpecialMarkets@reviewand
herald.com.

Autumn House® Publishing publishes biblically based materials for spiritual, physical, and mental growth and Christian discipleship.

The author assumes full responsibility for the accuracy of all facts and quotations as cited in
this book.

Unless otherwise noted, all Scripture passages are from the King James Version.

Texts credited to NIV are from the *Holy Bible, New International Version.* Copyright © 1973,
1978, 1984, International Bible Society. Used by permission of Zondervan Bible Publishers.
Texts credited to NKJV are from the New King James Version. Copyright © 1979,
1980, 1982, by Thomas Nelson, Inc. Used by permission. All rights reserved.
Scripture quotations marked NLT are taken from the *Holy Bible,* New Living
Translation, copyright © 1996. Used by permission of Tyndale House Publishers, Inc.,
Wheaton, Illinois 60189. All rights reserved.

This book was
Edited by Penny Estes Wheeler
Copyedited by James Cavil
Cover design by Ron Pride
Interior design by Candy Harvey
Cover photo by Traci Buck
Electronic makeup by Shirley M. Bolivar
Typeset: 12/14.5 Bembo

PRINTED IN U.S.A.
11 10 09 08 07   5 4 3 2 1

Library of Congress Cataloging-in-Publication Data
Sutton, Carolyn, 1944-   .
  Leaning on God's heart : when nothing is left, you still have God / Carolyn Sutton.
     p. cm.
  ISBN 978-0-8127-0433-4
  1. Consolation.   2. Suffering—Religious aspects—Christianity.   3. Spirituality.   I. Title.
  BV4909.S88 2007
  248.8'6—dc22

                    2006035116

DEDICATION

I gratefully dedicate this book to the
Creator, Sustainer, Sovereign,
and greatest love of my life—
my personal Physician—
Jesus Christ,
the Son of the living God,
on whose heart I am learning to lean.

In Special Recognition
of
Dr. Sandra Snyder

I didn't meet her before she was gone.
Yet, as with so many others,
during the brief time she had,
Sandra's faith, courage, love, and humor
touched my life, as well.
Someday soon
I plan to thank her . . .
in person.

CONTENTS

FOREWORD

Like Carolyn Sutton, I too am a cancer survivor—melanoma, fourth level. My spirit resonates with hers, and frankly I get a little choked up as she opens her heart in the pages of this book. Like Carolyn, I know what it feels like to "walk through the valley of the shadow of death." To stare at an uncertain future and exclaim, "O God! Why me?"

Tragically most advanced cancer patients don't have the luxury of sharing a testimony that resolves happily. For now, Carolyn and I do. Yet, as Carolyn so poignantly points out, we are all cancer survivors. We all reel from the physical, emotional, and spiritual side effects of the cancer of sin and its cruelty. Your cancer may not be intraductal carcinoma or non-Hodgkin's lymphoma. Rather, your "cancer" may be infertility. Or the aftermath of an abusive childhood. The death of a loved one. An eroding financial crisis. Divorce. Alzheimer's. Or the aging process.

Carolyn's diagnosis in this book correctly unwraps the Great Physician's Rx: God would have us focus on what lies beyond our "cancers." He is too wise to make a mistake and too good to be unkind. His heavenly medical advice is for us to go on with our lives—in His strength. To live them fully in Him.

With refreshing candor and humor, Carolyn frames her gripping story with ongoing reminders that only God can make a real difference—especially during times of physical and emotional crisis.

When all other supports fail, we can still know—as Carolyn's story reminds us—that "our darkest hour" can be "God's finest moment."[*] Anyone who reads this book will certainly find reassurance, encouragement, and hope for just one more day.

E. Lonnie Melashenko
Speaker/Director
Voice of Prophecy

---

[*] Mark M. Yarbrough, "When God Doesn't Heal," *Christianity Today*, September 2004, p. 80.

PREFACE

Did I *Really* Mean to Say That?

"Now there was leaning on Jesus' bosom one of his disciples, whom Jesus loved."
—*John 13:23*

I never thought I'd be writing a book about cancer—especially from a first-person perspective. Sure, as with most of us, a very remote possibility of my ever having cancer had crossed my mind. Yet, it did only once that I can recall—during the writing of my first book.[1]

In one paragraph I had praised God for his recent and obvious blessings in my life. Then I continued, "I have been learning to take nothing for granted. I take the joy as well as the growth in each 24-hour period." Almost as an aside, I added, "One of God's future goals for me may land me in the outback of Tasmania doing missionary work. Or perhaps three years from now I might best follow His will [by] sharing His good news with a fellow patient in some hospital cancer ward."[2]

After writing that last sentence, I remember pausing and asking myself, *Do I really mean that? Would I be courageous enough to stand by this statement if it should prove to be prophetic?* With a touch of spiritual bravado, perhaps, I left that sentence in the manuscript.

Seven years later I *did* become a patient in a hospital cancer ward (now referred to as an oncology unit). What I experienced during this unexpected journey through cancer I want to share with you. I want to share because, at one level or another, we are *all* dealing with "cancer," which threatens to eat away at our souls.

Your cancer may not be in the prostate or the breast or the liver or the lungs. No doctor may have given it a name, such as lymphoma or invasive ductal carcinoma or leukemia. A doctor hasn't had to name your cancer because you already know its name. Perhaps its name is fear . . . grief . . . irreversible diabetes . . . financial crisis . . . chemical imbalance disorder . . . aging . . .

11

divorce aftermath. . . estrangement from a child or a parent.

Whatever our cancers, they gnaw away at our vital energies and threaten to consume us.

On my journey through physical cancer, however, God gave me many opportunities to pause at what I'd call scenic viewpoints along the way. Pauses that afforded me time to reevaluate my perspectives regarding crisis and comfort, fear and faith, pain and praise.

Of course, I'll admit I'm a bit reluctant to walk back through these memories, revisiting places I would have chosen never to experience in the first place. Yet what I really want to share with you is the One who was already there in those dark places, waiting for me to show up, wild-eyed and shaken.

During my bout with cancer my neighbor Mary sent me an encouragement card. In it she extended this gracious invitation: *I'm praying for you. You can lean on my heart.* Throughout my journey through cancer I sensed God making me the same offer. He extends that offer to you as well.

How I learned to lean on His heart—in many different ways— is the theme of this book. For I've discovered that He has a habit of showing up at the midnight hour simply to listen, respond, and invite us to lean on His heart.

David often recognized the quiet arrival of Divinity. Of one occasion he wrote, "My heart has heard you [God] say, 'Come and talk with me.' And my heart responds, 'Lord, I am coming'" (Psalm 27:8, NLT).

No matter what our individual cancers, I pray that your experience and mine will be that of John the Beloved, who once described his tender relationship with Christ in these words: "Now there was *leaning on Jesus' bosom* one of his disciples, whom Jesus loved" (John 13:23).

May you and I learn to lean on the Son of God the way that John did. May we experience heart-to-heart intimacy with Divinity. During our souls' darkest nights, may His sustaining heartbeat perpetuate in us that refrain of constant renewal: "Yes, Jesus loves me!"

REMINDER
God invites us to lean on His heart,
especially during our darkest times.

MEDITATION
*"Come to me, all you who are weary and burdened,
and I will give you rest" (Matthew 11:28, NIV).*

---

[1] Carolyn Rathbun, *Journey to Joy: How God Can Fill the Empty Places of Your Heart* (Hagerstown, Md.: Review and Herald Pub. Assn., 1997). Available now only from the author (www.gracefulgrowthpresentations.org).

[2] *Ibid.,* p. 121.

Part I

A Darkening Storm

"I would hasten my escape from the windy storm and tempest."
—Psalm 55:8

In 2005 Hurricanes Katrina and Rita wreaked havoc in several Southern states, destroying homes, cities, and lives.

During this time people prayed—but the hurricane destroyed anyway. People began asking, "Where is God?" Have you noticed that we tend to raise this question more frequently in the face of a tragedy than on a day when the sun rises upon our well-ordered lives?

Because we live on a sin-infected planet, destructive storms often wreak havoc in our personal lives, leaving heartache, loss, and uncertainty in their wake. Some of us survive; some of us don't. More and more I'm realizing that survival is often a matter of choice—concerning the relationship we have with Someone.

Regarding these personal storm stories, I often reflect on a storm story from the Bible.

After a day of miracles, which included the feeding of far more than 5,000 hungry listeners, Jesus sent the people home (Matthew 14; Mark 6; John 6). Then He asked His disciples to get into their boat and sail across the Sea of Galilee toward Bethsaida.

The apostle John writes, "Then the sea arose because a great wind was blowing" (John 6:18, NKJV). The disciples wondered where Christ was, for John noted in his account of the story that Jesus hadn't yet come to them (verse 17).

Yet Mark (6:46) tells us *exactly* where Jesus was during the disciples' storm. He was up on the mountain praying for them. In addition to praying, He was doing something else. He was *watching* over them. "He [Jesus] saw that they [the disciples] were in serious trouble, rowing hard and struggling against the wind and waves" (verse 48, NLT).

Have you ever felt as if you were heading toward a God-appointed destination, your personal Bethsaida—traveling in a manner *He'd* ordained—only to have a sudden storm come up against you, maybe even blowing you off course? I'm sure you have, and so have I. During those times we too may be tempted, like John and the other disciples in that storm-battered ship, to ask, "Why hasn't He come to me?"

Gathering clouds

My journal entries the first few weeks of 2003 contained harbingers of a brewing storm that was about to unleash itself into my life and into the lives of those closest to me. A personal storm of hurricane proportions.

This book is that storm story, much of it told through journal entries that I kept during those months. Some of the chapters will relate "just the facts, ma'am." Others, however, will unfold in slow motion. For in them I wanted enough time together to remind of (1) who God is, (2) what His big plan for us entails, and (3) how much He wants us to lean on His heart in the midst of our storms. If we don't take time—habitually—to reflect on these three realities, our various cancers will consume both our spiritual and emotional health.

Cancer stories and victims seem to be coming out of the woodwork!

—Journal entry

The day ominous storm clouds formed on my personal horizon, I wrote my first journal entry with a pen—held in a slightly trembling hand.

January 6, 2003—*"Not a simple cyst." That's what my primary-care doctor said to me while looking over the ultrasound film.*

"This picture definitely reveals a mass that has changed size within the past three months. Let's have you checked out by a specialist."

What a way to start the new year!

16

January 7—*The receptionist at the specialist's office left a voice mail yesterday afternoon. The doctor can see me at 10:00 a.m. January 16. I've decided not to bother other family members or friends with this information until I know some facts. I'm trying to put this whole thing out of my mind until the sixteenth, but can think of little else.*

Tonight in our weekly Bible study the facilitator reminded us that we can know God's voice through His Word, the appeals of the Holy Spirit, and the unfolding of events in our everyday life. I wonder what God's about to say to me!

January 8—*Reported for county jury orientation today. The bailiff assigned me to a back pew in the first courtroom. We sat in silence, waiting. Then I started to notice those strange twinges in the area of that little lump on my left breast. To get my mind off of them, I closed my eyes to spend some of this dead time "in the secret place of the Most High." The bailiff said we'd be selected for jury duty today if our number comes up.*

In the context of this breast lump issue, I couldn't help wondering if my number is about to come up too or if I'll get off scot-free. In the courthouse my number never came up, and I was released to go home early. I hope that's a good omen.

Back home I e-mailed a couple of friends, asking them to quietly pray about my lump situation. I've decided to focus my time and energies on those closest to me and on tying up loose ends . . . just in case. I did an Internet search on breast cancer treatment today. Oooh! Depressing and frightening.

January 9—*No more being consumed by the consultation date! Today I choose to live each moment for the gift that it is. At 9:00 I'll walk with a friend. At 10:00 I'll proctor a midterm for a home school student. This afternoon I'll help my mother prepare her food for a birthday party with her grief recovery group—recently she's been handling Dad's death better. (I've been trying to do the same.) I sure wish Mom weren't blind, though. How life has closed in on her since losing her sight three and a half years ago!*

Tonight is my weekly date night with Jim. What a husband God found for me! I don't know whose turn it is to plan the date. If Jim can't remember either, I'll volunteer. I sure love him a lot—maybe I don't tell him enough.

January 10—*Mom phoned me tonight from her assisted living residence with a most extraordinary message. Regarding my possibly having cancer, she said, "I want you to know that whatever happens is all right with me. We must all die sometime. God is giving me an incredible peace about whichever one of us goes first. After all, this world is not our home." Bless you, sweet and strong mother!*

***January 11**—I am currently reading the autobiography of John Newton, author of "Amazing Grace." His wife died in the late 1700s of a "disease," as he refers to it—complications from a breast tumor the size of "half a melon."*

"If I make my bed in hell, behold, thou art there."

—Psalm 139:8

***January 13**—Cancer stories and victims seem to be coming out of the woodwork! While walking with my neighbor and new friend this morning, I was shocked when she shared with me that she's had two bouts with cancer. This vibrant, fast-paced woman is nearing the five-year cancer-free mark.*

Jim and I canned homemade applesauce today. Our apple tree really produced this year. The apples are organic—with a lot of worms! Working across the table from each other, we joked that we're hoping our bodies will be like the somewhat-misshapen apples with beautiful, healthy interiors (he has a prostate biopsy next week).

***January 16**—We met with the surgeon, who recommends an ultrasound needle biopsy on the mass in my left breast.*

***January 17**—I had another short night of sleep. Can't seem to drop off to sleep until I'm exhausted. I keep wondering if Jim has cancer . . . if we'll have to be apart while he's treated, so that Mother isn't left alone. He's my Rock of Gibraltar, my support, my love.*

Yet I'm Mother's rock. If I have cancer and have to undergo treatments that temporarily weaken me, there's no way I can care for her needs too. I feel so terribly torn.

Wait a minute! I don't even know the biopsy results yet, so I'm borrowing trouble. God, help me to trust in You. Help me to remember that nothing is a surprise to You and that You have promised to meet all our needs from Your own rich resources.

***January 18**—When I was pregnant, everyone else suddenly seemed pregnant too—I'd just never noticed before. Everywhere I looked I saw a pregnant woman. When I had back problems, people with back problems started coming out of the woodwork. Now I'm experiencing the same thing—*

but with cancer stories. At church today someone (who has no clue as to my current uncertainty) shared with me the story of a relative who had breast cancer. It seems as if the whole world has cancer!

January 20—*Jim had his biopsy today.*

January 22—*Today is the one-year anniversary of Mother's stroke. A year ago right now I was starting a three-day vigil with her at the local hospital. What a good year God has given her anyway!*

January 23—*Today Dr. Barrows' office phoned and told Jim he does not have prostate cancer! Half of my prayer has been answered as I wished it to be. If someone has to have cancer, I'd much rather that it be me. Thank You, God! Thank You!*

My doctor's office phoned to remind me of tomorrow's appointment when I'll get my biopsy results. My stomach is tight. I just have to remember that God is already in tomorrow.

REMINDER
Though life-changing storms come into every life,
Jesus, for whom no storm comes as a surprise,
is constantly watching over us.

༺༻

MEDITATION
" 'For I know the plans I have for you,' declares the Lord,
'plans to prosper you and not to harm you, plans to give you hope
and a future' " (Jeremiah 29:11, NIV).

Chapter 1

You Can't Go Back Again

"Things change. God doesn't."
—From a classroom poster

January 24, 2003—When I checked in at the surgeon's office, the receptionist pulled my file up. Clipped to the front was "Pathologist Report for Carolyn Sutton." I couldn't read upside down fast enough to get even a hint of what it said.

A few minutes later I tried not to flinch as the doctor reluctantly finished his sentence with "You have cancer." Those words would change my life forever. Nothing would ever be the same again.

I wanted to be strong for my husband. I prayed that I wouldn't cry. My arms went cold. My throat dried up.

The doctor continued as compassionately as he could. "Unfortunately, the pathologist's report shows your cancer type to be invasive lobular carcinoma. Also, the tumor is too large for you ever to be considered a cure. At best, you will be a survivor."

That's as good as it gets? This whole life-threatening scenario . . . just because of a little lump in my breast?

I suddenly remembered my maternal grandfather. He had died of cancer before I was even born. Several decades later one of his daughters, my aunt, fought colon cancer—and survived. Had I inherited cancer?

"Why?" I asked the doctor, trying to sound matter-of-fact.

"I can't tell you why," he said, shaking his head. "Your lifestyle would indicate that you shouldn't be a strong candidate at all for the disease."

Well, I shouldn't be, but evidently I was.

The doctor laid out treatment options, but oncology-speak was a whole new language to me. My mind just couldn't track. The doctor stood like a medical school lecturer beside his illuminated wall-mounted X-ray tray only a few feet away. Yet his voice sounded far off, as if I could barely hear it from the bottom of some deep, dark pit.

January 24 (continued)—At a restaurant an hour later I propped my elbow on the table while eating so that Jim wouldn't notice the wavy motion of the fork in my shaking hand. Jim commented, "I'm still in shock. It's like a bad dream that's not going to go away."

On the way home we stopped to share the disappointing news with Mother. She appeared to take it well and spoke of our needing to tap into strength and courage outside of ourselves. (She would certainly know about that!)

"I'm here for you no matter what," she emphasized. "And I love you so very much and am very, very proud of you. I know you'll handle this crisis in all the right ways." I thanked God that, in life at this point, I still had my mother's presence, strength, and wisdom.

We brought Mother home with us for the rest of the day. During this new journey the three of us would need one another more than ever.

January 25—Totally irrelevant nightmares punctuated my scant three hours of sleep last night. I spent my first waking hour in prayer and meditation. I'm glad that today is the Sabbath and that we're going to be visiting a little mountain church where no one has a clue what we're going through. "I will not leave you comfortless. . . . I . . . will manifest myself" [John 14:18-21] will be my banner text today.

At church Jim humbly yet eloquently shared his testimony. The Holy Spirit was palpable. Several people wept quietly as he spoke. I wept too. Part of the reason for my tears was an overwhelming fear about our uncertain future.

After the service I inquired about the pastor's absent wife. Her adult daughter told me the woman was home dealing with newly diagnosed cancer.

Dear God, I thought, *it's an epidemic!*

That evening Jim and I discussed treatment options. Whatever we chose as a treatment plan would have one overriding consideration: to stay ahead of death in this race—for as long as possible.

How can just one simple word, cancer, *bring all this upheaval and change into my life?* I wondered.

Life-changing words

Most of us have all heard shocking words that ushered in life transitions that would change our lives forever. A cancer diagnosis, in one way or another, that forced us to the end of our hope.

• Dorothy, I want a divorce.

• Mom, I'm pregnant.

• Sorry, Jessica, but in our latest downsize we have to phase out your job.

• Mrs. Smith, there's been an accident, and we need you to come to the morgue.

How *do* we cope with the aftermath of life-changing words? How do we deal with unwanted transition and change?

Perhaps the hardest aspect about irrevocable change is the terrible knowledge that we can't go back to the way things were.

A. W. Tozer once wrote, "The man with a cross no longer controls his own destiny; he lost control when he picked up the cross. That cross immediately became to him an all-absorbing interest, an overwhelming interference." [1]

The three-legged stool

Three realizations during the early part of my journey through cancer held me up like three legs on a little stool.

The first leg of my spiritual stool was simply to surrender to the spiritual reality that *God knows best.* Bible passages such as Romans 11:33-36 reminded me that God alone has the wisdom concerning what to allow or not allow into our lives. "For who hath known the mind of the Lord?" Paul asked (Romans 11:34).

The prophet Daniel cautions us mere mortals that we really

don't have the wisdom to hurl at God a "What are You doing?" challenge (see Daniel 4:35). God alone is all-knowing.

Fellow travelers who grew . . . anyway

As I struggled to keep my emotional head above water in the aftermath of the earthshaking cancer diagnosis, I also took strength from those who had walked this path before me: those who had done so while still clinging to their belief that God is good—all the time. That was the second leg of my spiritual stool.

"A little leaven leaveneth the whole lump."

—Galatians 5:9

John Newton, the eighteenth-century former slave trader and born-again man of God, lost his wife to complications from a very large breast tumor. Yet so completely submitted to God's sovereignty was Newton that he had absolutely *no* desire to go back to the way things had been, as evidenced in the following words.

"He [God] had loaned her [my wife] to me," Newton wrote, "and He who loaned her had a right to take her back when He chose. Had He given me what I deserved, He would have taken her back the first day I got her. I was just thankful I'd had her so long."[2]

Newton added, "His sovereignty is connected to His infinite wisdom and goodness. If it were possible for me to alter any part of His plan, I could only spoil it."[3]

Amazing!

Prayer therapy

The third supportive leg of my spiritual stool during the early stages of my journey was my knowing that I could talk to God about the unsettling changes going on in my life.

Author Mike Mason states that "what distinguishes [Job] from his friends is his ability to live with the awful untenableness of his situation. He does not like it; he does not understand it. But somehow in the midst of it he manages to hold himself together like the driver of a team of wild horses. . . . Job is out of control and knows it, and so calls desperately upon the Lord to take the reins."[4]

King David said, "Blessed be the Lord, because he hath heard the voice of my supplications. The Lord is my strength and my shield; my heart trusted in him, and I am helped: therefore my heart greatly rejoiceth" (Psalm 28:6, 7).

Not long after my cancer diagnosis, I phoned the local bank with a question about our check order. The woman at the other end of the line picked up the receiver and cheerfully greeted me with these words: "Thanks for calling the world's greatest bank! How may I help you?"

I loved it!

"For if the firstfruit be holy, the lump is also holy."

—Romans 11:16

Yet her enthusiastic response is but a dim reflection of the enthusiasm with which God embraces our prayers. After all, isn't heaven the universe's greatest bank of spiritual blessings? Blessings that God is more than willing to bestow upon us when we answer His ever-ready question to us, "How may I help you?"

E. M. Bounds points out that the answers to our prayers rest not only on God's promises, but also upon our relationship to Him as one of His children.[5] So as I talk to God about life's dark surprises, I am learning to lean on the strength of my *Father*.

Facing the future

When a cancer keeps us from going back to the way that things were before, we are actually in some very distinguished company spiritually.

Joseph, after being sold to Arabian slave traders, could never go back again.

Daniel, after being captured and emasculated by the Babylonians, could never go back again.

John the Beloved, exiled to the bleak isle of Patmos, could never go back again.

Each one of these men faced some type of "cancer." Yet look at how God worked in their lives—precisely *because* they couldn't go back again.

Joseph helped to rescue the Egyptian civilization from starvation, and saved his own family in the process. Through Joseph's cancer of exile, God established the nation of Israel.

While in captivity Daniel received a prophetic ministry from God. The angel Gabriel appeared, called him "greatly beloved," (Daniel 9:23-27), and then gave him the "crown jewels" of Old Testament prophecy.[6]

In vision John saw the New Jerusalem. His description of its astounding beauty has offered eternal hope to millions.

In a sense Joseph, Daniel, and John were truly cancer survivors—*spiritual* survivors, that is. We can become spiritual survivors as well—even if we can't go back again. While acknowledging our fear of the unknown, we can simultaneously secure our position on the three-legged stool and face the future with God.

After all, if God has an ongoing plan for my life and if crisis is part of that plan, why should I cling to the past and the way things were?

January 26—Our bluegrass music group went this evening to audition for the local school's upcoming talent show. Ah, musical therapy. "Keep on the sunny side!" the little hammers pounded out on my dulcimer. Lord, help me internalize those words.

January 28—I've been using part of my devotional time keying Bible promises and hymns into the computer. As of this morning I'm starting my personal devotions with an out-loud hymn of praise. My voice is sounding shaky, but I want to hear myself entoning words of hope and faith. I want God to hear them too (not to mention the enemy who wants to take me out).

I know I can't ever go back again to the way things were before my cancer diagnosis. So the first line of today's hymn is "Anywhere with Jesus I can safely go." Lord, now as never before, help me accept the truth behind the words of that song!

REMINDER

We lean on God's heart when we sit securely on the three-legged spiritual stool He has provided us: (1) His omniscience; (2) the encouraging examples of other survivors; and (3) God's accessibility through our prayers.

⊙

MEDITATION

"These things happened to them as examples and were written down as warnings for us, on whom the fulfillment of the ages has come. . . . No temptation has seized you except what is common to man. And God is faithful; he will not let you be tempted beyond what you can bear. But when you are tempted, he will also provide a way out so that you can stand up under it" *(1 Corinthians 10:11-13, NIV).*

---

[1] A. W. Tozer, "True Faith Must Influence Our Daily Living," *Renewed Day by Day,* ed. F. B. Smith (Harrisburg, Pa.: Christian Publications, 1980). As quoted in David Biebel, *If God Is So Good, Why Do I Hurt So Bad?* (Grand Rapids: Fleming H. Revell, 1989), p. 88.

[2] John Newton, in *John Newton, Letters of a Slave Trader Freed by God's Grace,* par. Dick Bohrer (Chicago: Moody Press, 1983), p. 118.

[3] *Ibid.*

[4] Mike Mason, *The Gospel According to Job* (Wheaton, Ill.: Crossway Books, 1994), p. 134.

[5] E. M. Bounds, *The Complete Works of E. M. Bounds on Prayer* (Peabody, Mass.: Prince Press, 1990), p. 239.

[6] Gerhard Pfandl, "Daniel," *Adult Sabbath School Bible Study Guide,* October-December 2004, p. 88.

Chapter 2

Why? And Other Questions Cancer Makes You Ask

"Much of the dialogue in Job illustrates the exasperating paradox that when life is good we tend to have no questions, but when life is bad we have no answers."
—Mike Mason[1]

January 27, 2003—I had to break the news by phone to two more friends today. The fact that nobody cried (for a change) was helpful, though the unspoken pain was palpable.

Earlier today, while we were cleaning out the freezer, Jim and I kept falling into each other's arms and weeping. We kept telling each other, "It's going to be OK because God is in control." Yet we both understand that God's definition of OK may not be our definition of OK.

I'd almost forgotten that emotional suffering can be almost as intense as physical suffering. These recurring questions overwhelm me. I wish I had the answers!

During traumatizing crisis we find ourselves asking questions about our loss or setback. We're equally as serious about finding *answers* that can help us make sense of our cancer.

Although your cancer and mine may not be the same, perhaps you can relate to some of the questions my disease made me ask. In particular I grappled with three questions: First, why this setback in *my* life? Next, is what's happening to me my fault? And third, can there be any *purpose* for a seemingly senseless cancer like this?

We'll deal with the first of these questions now, and the last two in the next chapter.

Though I won't have all the answers to my question until God gives them to me on the other side (see Deuteronomy 29:29), here are some of the thought processes through which my answer-seeking led me.

Question 1: Why this kind of setback in my life? (also known as the "Why *me?*" question)

For several days following my cancer diagnosis I grappled with this, the most predominant, question: Why me? Yet the longer I mulled it over, the more it changed shape. Eventually "Why me?" metamorphosed into *Whatever made me think I have the right to expect a trouble-free life?* Since when did I assume such a state of entitlement that I deserve to be exempt from tragedy and hardship while everyone else in the world suffers?

The answer is that I *don't* deserve to be exempt. I'll never be exempt this side of eternity, because I'm a member of the human race. A race living on a planet that is under the dominion of one who is intent on destroying us (as God Himself unveiled in Job 2:3).

Because the enemy of our souls seeks as a roaring lion to devour us (1 Peter 5:8), you and I will suffer loss and pain and trial. Therefore, we shouldn't be shocked (though we usually are) when trouble comes.

While groping to make sense out of my cancer diagnosis, I began noticing more subtleties in my Bible reading. For example, God, through Isaiah, said, "When you pass through the waters, I will be with you. . . . When you walk through the fire, you will not be burned" (Isaiah 43:2, NIV).

Notice that God didn't say, "*If* you pass through the waters or walk through the fire." He said *when*.

Sooner or later we all experience cancer in our lives. The Ecclesiast warned that in this life we all will experience "a time to weep" as well as "a time to mourn," and "a time to lose" (see Ecclesiastes 3:4, 6)—probably many times over.

Back to Why me?

As I reflected on my diagnosis, I realized all the times in life when I didn't bother to ask, "Why me?"

28

I didn't ask "Why me?" when I gave birth to a *healthy* baby boy, despite the fact that he arrived five weeks early. Two hardworking Catholic nuns in a little African jungle hospital delivered him during a mission generator failure, with the aid of a flashlight and a kerosene lantern as their only light sources.

Years later I didn't ask "Why me?" when this only child chose to stay away from drugs, working hard to obtain higher education in preparation for a career helping troubled kids.

I didn't ask "Why me?" when God brought a beautiful husband into my life several years after a devastating divorce. I never questioned why God allowed my loving parents' presence in my life until I was almost 60 years old. And I don't remember crying out "Why me?" whenever a little royalty check from my writing endeavors arrived in the mail.

Considering all these blessings, I suddenly wondered, *What right do I have to complain when storms blow into my life? Even when they blow me off course on my way toward Bethsaida!*

What good does a knowledge of God do for me when I'm facing tough stuff that may never go away?

Job asked, "Shall we indeed accept good from God, and shall we not accept adversity?" (Job 2:10, NKJV). If Job could make that statement in the midst of everything he endured, what was *my* problem?

How often we overlook the reality that God is sovereign (Psalm 115:3). Therefore, He is under no obligation to fulfill our every desire concerning what He does—or doesn't—allow into our lives.

With shame I realized my false assumption that living conscientiously would somehow—and always—put me beyond the reach of serious disease—or other personal crises. What arrogance! I decided.

January 30—*I just wish this whole rotten cancer thing would simply go away!*

"On the other hand," as a friend of mine often says, I *do* have a perfect right in times of shock, uncertainty, grief, and fear to give honest expression to my emotions. After all, God created me to have feelings.

When I react emotionally to a personal crisis, I'm in distinguished company. Joseph wept loudly when he saw his brothers after many years of separation. David and Jonathan grieved deeply upon saying goodbye to each other for the last time. So did Naomi when she parted with her daughter-in-law Orpah.

And then we remember Job's emotional outburst when he exclaimed, "I loathe my life. . . . Let me alone" (Job 7:16, NKJV).

One of my favorite authors, Ellen Gould White, also gave honest expression to her feelings in times of discouragement, as evidenced by the following journal entries.

May 19, 1859—*"Miserable in health and depressed in spirits. . . . Oh, how desolate my heart feels! A strange sadness is upon me. I am so lonely, so distressed! Such a gloom rests upon everything. It seems that a heavy stone is placed upon my heart. O God, do not forsake me in my weakness and misery.*

"I sometimes think that my work is done, and feelings come over me that I am of no use, can do no good; and then it seems as though it would be a sweet relief to rest in the grave."

May 20, 1859—*"Disease is bearing me down. My heavenly Father alone knows my almost constant pain. I have found relief in prayer today. It did seem that the Lord heard me and would pity me. I am sorry I feel so deeply and am so sensitive. But few can enter into or understand my feelings or trials. But God knows all. He is acquainted with the whole burdened heart. May the Lord be pleased to revive my courage and lift up my desponding heart and water it with the dew of heaven, that it may flourish again."* [2]

Finally, our most precious comrade in suffering is Jesus. In the Garden of Gethsemane, in unspeakable anguish, Christ sweat great drops of blood as humanity's sins weighed upon Him and a sense of impending separation from God overwhelmed Him.

This side of heaven we may never know *why* particular storms blow into our lives. And no matter what anyone else says or thinks, we *do* have a right to grieve them. Expressing our emotions is part of what makes us human—as Christ Himself demonstrated when He lived among us.

Managing our feelings

I notice a common thread running through the experiences of the individuals mentioned above. They accepted the reality of their personal crises. Although they honestly expressed their emotions, they also *managed* them. They did not allow overwhelming emotion to keep them from moving ahead with life.

Amy Givler, medical doctor and cancer survivor, expresses in *Hope in the Face of Cancer* the wide emotional range she experienced: timidity, shame, guilt, withdrawal, anxiety, and fatigue.

Dr. Givler cautions, however, that we can't let emotions get in the way of our decision-making. This includes the emotions of other people. She writes, "The sooner I can accept this new and unpleasant reality of cancer, the sooner I can fight it with all of my strength."[3]

I believe that when we allow God to enable our acceptance of sin's cancer in our lives, we can continue the good fight, under His watchful eye—even if we're still asking why.

After all, even on the cross, that is what Jesus did (Mark 15:34).

REMINDER

We lean on God's heart when we let Him strengthen us for the fight, even when we don't know all the answers.

MEDITATION

"My eyes fail from weeping, I am in torment within, my heart is poured out on the ground." "Because of the Lord's great love we are not consumed, for his compassions never fail. They are new every morning; great is your faithfulness" (Lamentations 2:11; 3:22, 23, NIV).

---

[1] Mike Mason, *The Gospel According to Job,* p. 141.

[2] Ellen G. White manuscript 6, 1859.

[3] Amy Givler, M.D., *Hope in the Face of Cancer: A Survival Guide for the Journey You Did Not Choose* (Eugene, Oreg.: Harvest House Publishers, 2003), p. 43.

Chapter 3

The Only Real Answer . . . for Now

"I don't shake my fist at the heavens anymore, and I don't ask why.
Life is too short to search for answers that may or may not exist;
some days are just plain tough and there's no getting around them."
—Janet Dagon[1]

March 22, 2003 (Jim's and my sixth wedding anniversary)—*I turned out the light and rolled over on my side. Silently I cried out, "Precious Jesus, if this is what it takes to purify my life, then so be it. Just be with me, comfort me, and put Your healing hand on me—whatever that means to You." I tried to visualize myself resting in His arms and His understanding the pain I couldn't.*

In the previous chapter we concluded that although this side of heaven we may not know why we go through certain trials, we can still allow them to help strengthen our faith in God.

Let's look at the second of the three questions we posed: Is what's happening to me my fault?

In other words: *Am I to blame for my cancer?*

My mind grew exhausted as I rehearsed again and again my personal risk factors. Heredity. Lifestyle. Nutrition habits. Stress in recent years. Medications taken, and abandoned.

I also rehearsed what I believed I'd done right—and wrong (even if done innocently, such as relying on long-ago medical counsel before practitioners knew what they now know about the harmful side effects of certain medications).

In addition to my fears over the unexpected cancer diagnosis, I began assigning blame. If only my ancestors hadn't had cancer . . . if only I hadn't been on the Pill so long . . . if only I hadn't lost so much sleep all those years I was teaching . . . if only I'd been more careful about fat in my diet . . . if only I'd been more assertive when that first specialist didn't acknowledge my concerns about that second little lump—the malignant one—in my breast.

Author Mason states, "Surely this is the hardest part of any suffering: trying to decide whether this is an undeserved attack that the Lord has allowed for the sake of His own glory, or whether it is something we have brought upon ourselves through sin and foolishness."[2]

For a time the if-onlys threatened to consume me just as they did the children of Israel. Though the Israelites should have assumed the blame they sometimes directed toward Moses and Aaron, way too frequently they focused on the if-onlys from their past.

"If only we'd stayed in Egypt. If only we'd died in the desert" (see Numbers 14:2). Their regret over not being able to change things in the past undermined the trust they should have had in God for their present.

I realized that if I weren't careful I could fall into the same trap. Of course, some of the blame I did assign to myself. However, the if-onlys of the past could *not* help me in the present. Why waste good emotional energy on things from the past over which I may or may not have had control? The only control I now had over my if-onlys was to give them to God.

I finally did.

The children of Israel also experienced *fear* concerning their future. They feared what Canaan's giants might do to them tomorrow (Numbers 13:30–14:5), thereby lacking heart to take possession of the Promised Land *today*. Likewise, I feared the giants.

I feared that when word got out about my cancer, others might judge me as being responsible for it. I feared some might interrogate me about my personal habits, find fault with them, and then blame me (rightly or wrongly) for bringing this disease upon myself.[3]

Lifestyle choices *do* have a tremendous and direct impact on the quality of one's health. Yet the story of Job reminds us that in a sinful world, holy doesn't *always* equal healthy. Factors of which we are ignorant may also be in play. The apostle Peter pointed out that we sometimes criticize and judge what—or whom—we do not understand (2 Peter 2:12).

Someone once stated that believing that we get what we earn from our righteous living can be ruinous to our faith. Most of us know individuals who have lost faith in God when their prayers weren't answered according to their desires. One woman told me, "I just don't get why God didn't answer my prayers when I'd been trying so hard to do everything right!"

Feeling betrayed, the woman allowed her disappointment and anger with God to replace her faith in Him.

To be perfectly honest . . .

Since I'm trying to tell my cancer story frankly, I'll share something God pointed out to me regarding *my* fear of being criticized and judged. What I feared from others were the same critical attitudes *I* had held in the past toward certain individuals with health problems. Individuals whom I had judged from within the privacy of my own sinful soul.

Ouch, God! And thank You.

Of a grave illness that once befell him, John Newton wrote, "I fell sick with a high fever that put me flat on my back, *where God could reach me.*"[4]

Solomon accurately observed, "Blows that hurt cleanse away evil, as do stripes the inner depths of the heart" (Proverbs 20:30, NKJV; see also Job 23:10 and 1 Peter 1:7).

> *"Fear none of those things which thou shalt suffer . . . that ye may be tried; . . . be thou faithful . . ."*
> —Revelation 2:10

Once I realized judgmentalism as one of *my* sins, I asked God to forgive me for jumping to uninformed conclusions about people on whom I had passed hasty judgment—when the reasons for their problems were definitely none of *my* business.

Humbled, I gave God the giants of tomorrow to put with yesterday's if-onlys, so I could focus on how He wanted me to proceed *today*.

And now the third question: Can there be any *purpose* for such a seemingly senseless cancer as this?

The *Big* Why?

If anyone ever walked by faith and leaned on God's heart in the process, it was Moses. Yet guess what? Moses asked God, "Why?" (Exodus 5:22).

So can you and I. Not that God has promised to tell us all the answers to our every "Why?" mind you. No, He never promised to do that. (Again, we can refer to Deuteronomy 29:29.)

However, God did tell us that our "steps are directed by the Lord. How then can anyone understand his own way?" (Proverbs 20:24, NIV).

We can't. Yet Hebrews 12:1, 2 does suggest that our suffering has a purpose that we will understand in God's own time—whether that's the day after tomorrow or 30,000 eons from now.

Through His Word God has given us sort of a multiple-choice answer sheet regarding the great Why questions we often ask Him. So let's consider them for the question "What could possibly be the purpose for my current cancer?"

Option A: The purpose of my cancer is to test my faith.

Psalm 11:5 states that God allows tests to come to His children. Revelation 2:10 states, "Fear none of those things which thou shalt suffer: behold, the devil shall cast some of you into prison, that ye may be tried." Perhaps current suffering is a test, which will serve to strengthen faith in God.

When you think about it, no biblical giant (man or woman) and no Hebrews 11 hero avoided a fiery trial.

A flood swept away Noah's world.

A military leader forced Deborah to go to war.

Religious zealots stoned Stephen.

Herod beheaded John the Baptist.

Fear made Jonah run away from ministry before finally embracing it.

God forbade Jeremiah to marry before he was beaten, thrown into a slimy pit, then forced into exile—by his *own* countrymen!

Today you and I, among millions who read the Bible, can look to these survivors for courage and reassurance to strengthen our faith (Romans 10:17).

Perhaps you and I, just as they, are being tested during this journey through our trials. Who is watching us? Who will gain comfort and encouragement—and have strengthened faith—from our God-centered response to suffering?

Option B: The purpose of our cancer is to make a positive life change . . . for eternity.

Another purpose for our cancers may be that something in our lives needs changing in order for God to save us.

Take Peter, for instance.

Peter failed his great test on the eve of the Crucifixion by denying Christ. This failure was the beginning of a new conversion experience that changed his self-confident pride into humility (John 21:15-19).

Then there was Job.

Though he was a man God described as perfect, Job still had self-justifying tendencies (Job 29-31). By the end of Job's trials, however, his focus had shifted from his own good works to God and God alone (Job 42:6).

More important to God than seeing us through our temporal cancers is saving us for His eternal kingdom. Perhaps that's why He promised in Revelation 2:10 that if—in our trials—we are "faithful unto death," He will give us "a crown of life."

Option C: The purpose of my cancer is to help me know God better.

I spent the first 17 years of my life living on campuses of boarding schools. Both my parents were educators. When I was in the sixth grade, Mrs. Lorenz, a new girls' physical education teacher, joined the high school staff. To me she seemed very serious, even unapproachable. Whenever she was on chaperone duty during the Saturday night sports/roller skating activities in the gymnasium, I steered clear of her.

One Saturday night I was skate-racing with my girlfriends on the wooden floor of the gym. Round the basketball court we flew. I suddenly saw my opening to get ahead of the others, and leaned to an inside lane to pass Nancy.

Suddenly my right skate jerked to a standstill, stopped by an un-tied skate lace that quickly wound about the axle of a wheel. In a heartbeat I flew through the air and landed hard on my bare knees. The momentum skidded me across the floor.

I don't know what hurt worse—my burning skin-peeled knees or my pride. On my side, I writhed in pain. Blood streaming from my knees quickly puddled on the floor. As one of the activity chap-erones blew his whistle, signaling the other skaters to clear the floor, I suddenly felt a comforting hand on my shoulder.

"Let's get you patched up," a kind voice said. I looked up to see Mrs. Lorenz leaning over me. Gently she helped me to my feet, took off my skates, and replaced them with my shoes. With tissues she dabbed at the blood freely oozing from my knees and soaking the top of my bobby socks.

Slowly she walked me up the hill to the duplex where she and her husband lived. After having me sit on the side of their bathtub, Mrs. Lorenz poured hydrogen peroxide over my knees and gently bathed the blood from my legs.

I couldn't believe this was the same teacher I had feared so much. Precisely because of my skating de-bacle I was now experiencing traits of hers that I never would have imagined. From then on, Mrs. Lorenz became my hero, my role model, and one of my all-time favorite teachers.

"My purpose is to know God, to please Him, to be found faithful to Him, and even to be known as His friend."

—David Biebel [5]

When we let God take care of us in the midst of our crises, we will experience Him in ways we never before thought possible.

Multiple-choice answers

Let's return to the question before us: What could possibly be the purpose for our current cancer?

A. To test our faith.

B. To change our lives for eternity.

C. To help us know God better.

I wouldn't be surprised if on God's multiple-choice answer sheet

He had two more options:

D. All of the above.

E. So much more . . . than all the above! (See Ephesians 3:20.)

Before I finished my journey through cancer, I began to strongly suspect that options A through E were *all* part of the answer to the biggest "Why?" question I'd ever had.

In the words of one cancer survivor, *"Why* is not the question. Rather, *trust* is the answer."[6]

REMINDER

We lean on God's heart when we trust Him with today—
leaving both yesterday and tomorrow in His capable hands.

MEDITATION

"Therefore do not worry about tomorrow, for tomorrow will worry about itself. Each day has enough trouble of its own" (Matthew 6:34, NIV).

[1] Janet Dagon, in *Adventist Review,* May 23, 1991.

[2] I'm grateful to share that this fear was most ungrounded in my case. I experienced nothing but prayer support, compassion, and nonjudgmentalism on all sides.

[3] Mike Mason, *The Gospel According to Job,* p. 238.

[4] John Newton, in *John Newton, Letters of a Slave Trader,* p. 73.

[5] David Biebel, *If God Is So Good, Why Do I Hurt So Bad?* p. 170.

[6] From Pastor Don Livesay's cancer journey testimony shared publicly at a July 2003 camp meeting in Gladstone, Oregon.

Chapter 4

What Next, Coach?

Now it's time to read and pray and cry and gather strength for today—
as I begin what is certain to be a long, painful journey into the unknown.
I've asked the pastor for anointing after prayer meeting this week.
I want God to be at the head of this whole operation.
—Journal entry

W hat next, Coach?"
That's an expression my husband uses when he comes up against a brick wall. Sometimes he also addresses this question to me when he wants my input on something. I even ask Jim this same question now when I'm in a quandary about a decision I need to make.

Sometimes, however, the only coach we can turn to is God.

That was certainly the situation when Jim and I realized we'd need to make some treatment choices concerning my cancer—and quickly. Deciding on a cancer treatment plan was one of the most agonizing decisions of my adult life. After heart-searching prayer, after personal research in books and on the Internet, and after much counseling, my family and I settled on a blend of treatment modalities—both natural and medical.[1]

Yet before we began treatment, I first wanted to allow God the opportunity to do whatever He saw fit regarding my cancer.

January 27, 2003—I've asked our pastor for a private, quiet anointing after prayer meeting tomorrow evening at the church. Since anointing is a strong biblical recommendation, I want this step to be a first resort—not a last one—before I start the actual treatment process.

What it means to be anointed

I requested anointing . . . with oil in the name of the Lord (see James 5:14) to fulfill my heart's desire that the accompanying "prayer of faith" should "save the sick, and the Lord shall raise [her, in my case] up" (verse 15).

Yet I wanted to be careful not to *demand* divine healing. After all, when God granted the insistent requests of the Israelites, He also read "sent leanness into their soul" (Psalm 106:15, NKJV). The NIV rendition of this verse states that God sent "a wasting disease upon them." I certainly didn't want answered prayer—even if it meant healing—to be at the expense of a diseased soul.

So what does it really mean to be anointed? I wondered. I did a little search and came up with the following biblical information.

To be anointed means to be set aside for a special purpose (Exodus 30:26-30; Numbers 7:1). Anointing also infers the bestowal of the Holy Spirit (Isaiah 61:1). Paul wrote, "Now He who establishes us with you in Christ and has anointed us is God, who also has sealed us and given us the Spirit in our hearts as a guarantee" (2 Corinthians 1:21, 22, NKJV).

Above all, I craved the cleansing power of the Holy Spirit in my life, which is the second part of the promise about anointing given in James 5:15—"and if he have committed sins, they shall be forgiven him."

Certainly I wanted to be made right with God.

Researching further, I discovered that David, when afflicted and in pain, wanted—more than anything—for his sins to be forgiven. "Look upon mine affliction and my pain; and forgive all my sins" (Psalm 25:18). He affirmed that God "is the saving refuge of His anointed" (Psalm 28:8, NKJV).

In Paul's words, I too wanted God to free me from "the power of darkness." I wanted Him to convey me "into the kingdom of the Son of His love, in whom we have redemption through His blood, the forgiveness of sins" (Colossians 1:13, 14, NKJV).

As the date of my anointing approached, I went on a prayerful heart and memory search.

Taking care of business

January 27 (continued)—I've been doing the work of heart searching and confession in preparation [for anointing]. I even wrote someone a letter today regarding an incident that took place 37 years ago. One of my close friends thought the matter too trivial to merit a letter, but I wanted to remove all doubt in my mind.

And searching my heart, I discovered some unfinished business. I sought out the location of an old boyfriend and sent an e-mail to his workplace. Here is an excerpt from my note.

Dear Henry,[2]

I hope this e-note finds you and yours doing well. . . . Congratulations on your professional achievements!

[In addition to other responsibilities at this point in my life] I also teach a youth class at our little church. A while back the kids and I were discussing the necessity of asking forgiveness when we have hurt people in some way. I recalled—as I have a number of times throughout the years—how one of my choices hurt you.

[During our] senior class trip you pushed me into the river one evening just after I'd showered and done my hair. I was offended and hurt because you seemed to think it was a joke. [Back at school] the following Friday, in order to playfully "get even," I asked a friend of my brother's to let the air out of one of the back tires of your car that you always parked outside the cafeteria. I thought it was funny and was going to "fess up" that day. I thought you'd think it was funny too.

You phoned later that weekend to tell me you suspected that someone was out to get you because they'd let the air out of your tire. You were very distraught and had been late to work because of the flat tire [for which I'd been responsible!]. Not wanting to incur your anger, I decided to wait a bit before admitting the truth. The perfect time to confess what I'd done never seemed to come before we eventually parted ways. The reality is that I was just a big coward.

Although you might not remember this incident, I do. I also remember that during those years you were still dealing with the aftermath of your father's death and also the loss of another close family member. What I had

*done to your tire was unwarranted, vindictive, and selfish. I'm ashamed of
it and ask your forgiveness.*

Warm regards.

Nine days later my former boyfriend sent me a reply. Here are
some excerpts.

Dear Carolyn,

*Your e-mail was quite unexpected but did paint a smile on my face. To
be honest, the particular circumstance that you referenced is beyond my recall.*

*As for the forgiveness part, that is not a problem. You are forgiven. In
fact, I am probably in "need" of forgiveness for things that I did or said but
now do not recall (dementia can be our friend if we can just remember to let
it do the job).*

Then after catching me up on highlights of his life, he closed
with *Good to hear from you, Henry.*

Maybe God allowed cancer to invade my body so that I would
finally allow Him to treat a spiritual disease eating away at my right-
ful place in the kingdom. Perhaps He was graciously giving me the
opportunity to trust the promise of 1 John 1:9, enabling me to claim
forgiveness for an unconfessed sin I had let slide for nearly 40 years!

Another ugliness that God pointed out in my heart was spiritual
pride. I'd been tempted to think that my "goodness" in lifestyle
habits should have kept me from having cancer. "Of all people," said
one friend, "this shouldn't happen to you. You're faithful about exercise. You don't eat—" And on she went. Her comments felt good,
and inwardly I agreed. Yet my response to these words smacked of
salvation by works. Again I asked God's forgiveness.

What a loving God He is to lead us in ways and by means that
will work not only for His glory but also for our eternal good!

As Joni Earickson Tada once emphasized in a television interview, God's primary focus is to prepare us for eternity. Nothing else
about us matters more to Him.

In her interview Tada pointed out a telling incident in the

Gospel of Mark. When Peter and other disciples came searching for Christ early one Sunday morning to persuade Him to return to the village, Christ answered in these words: "Let us go into the next towns, that I may preach there also, because *for this purpose* I have come forth" (Mark 1:38, NKJV).

Friday, January 31—*The anointing service was in the primary/junior room two days ago. The pastor, Jim, and three other elders were present. I asked to share for a few minutes—about the history of cancer in my family, about why I've chosen the treatment modalities I have, and about the condition of my faith at this point. Jim read a couple of encouraging thoughts. Then each person present prayed over me. It was a tearful time for all of us. Yet it was a precious time. (How my heart breaks for Jim!)*

During the anointing service that Wednesday night my brothers in Christ placed their hands on me. The pastor touched oil to my forehead and prayed.

Was I miraculously healed of my cancer?

No.

Were my sins forgiven followed by the most cleansing sense of peace I've ever experienced?

Yes. A thousand times . . . *yes!*

Life after cancer would never the same, it's true. Happily, neither would life after anointing.

REMINDER

More than wanting us to have healthy bodies, God wants us to have healthy souls.

MEDITATION

"Now I know that the Lord saves His anointed; He will answer [her] from His holy heaven with the saving strength of His right hand"
(Psalm 20:6, NKJV).

---

[1] A cautionary word: I am purposely not sharing in this book why I chose the treatment modalities that I did. I wouldn't want anyone to read what I did and think, *Well, that seemed to have worked for her, so maybe I'll do that too.*

In my personal research I learned that "there are more than a hundred different cancers, each with teams of information available about it—who is at risk for getting it, what it acts like, and how it's treated" (Amy Givler, *Hope in the Face of Cancer,* p. 88). Anyone with a cancer diagnosis needs to *prayerfully* make his or her own *informed* decision about treatment.

Yes, I believe with *all* my heart that many people have been healed through natural treatment methods alone. Others have experienced apparent healing through the traditional medical modalities, though with the ongoing aftermath of lingering side effects, to be sure. Yet the grim statistics on this sin-ridden planet reveal death in both camps.

All I will say about my treatment choices is this: my family and I made our decisions only after several weeks of intense prayer. During this time we also took counsel with medical, wholistic, and lay practitioners as well as with cancer survivors. We did research in medical books, research in spiritual books, and research on the Internet.

We read specifically about my type of cancer and looked at it from as many perspectives as we could: cancer type, tumor size, whether it was estrogen/progesterone receptive/negative, and so on. We also watched unfolding events in our lives and waited for the voice of the Spirit.

In the end, we followed what we believed to be God's unmistakable guidance for me in my situation . . . but not necessarily for you in yours!

[2] Not his real name.

Chapter 5

New Scars and Old

"Character cannot be developed in ease and quiet. Only through experience of trial and suffering can the soul be strengthened, ambition inspired, and success achieved."
—Attributed to Helen Keller

How quickly the final days of January passed!
I found myself wanting to disassociate from my health crisis. After cancer's initial exposure, however, the disease doesn't politely stop spreading in order that its victim have time to work through the shock of diagnosis . . . or help family and friends adjust . . . or become philosophical about this dark surprise.

Sooner or later (preferably sooner) the cancer survivor must implement a chosen plan—before it's too late. For me that time was rapidly approaching.

Yes, I trusted that God was watching over me. Yes, I was sitting on my "spiritual stool." Yes, I had resolved to trust God come what may. I'd even chosen a theme text for this journey: "The joy of the Lord is your strength" (Nehemiah 8:10, NIV). I'd also prayerfully put together a treatment plan. However, it was time to *implement* the plan on which I'd prayerfully decided.

The plan was as follows:

Ongoing treatment: as much fresh and raw foods in my diet as possible, a certain amount of juicing, continuing outdoor exercise, copious amounts of water, and selected natural supplements.

Short-term treatment: a lumpectomy (versus mastectomy), possibly chemotherapy, and maybe radiation. In the three weeks preceding my surgery, I went to work on a writing project. A year or so earlier I'd put it on a back burner because of Mom's growing health concerns and her need for me to be more available to her.

Aware that my upcoming surgical procedure entailed routine risks, I now decided to finish the project—in my "spare" time—before cancer treatment began. So at a time when my life felt completely off-kilter, I completed the manuscript and submitted it to a publisher. Ironically, the theme of the manuscript was . . . how to obtain and maintain personal balance!*

February 4, 2003 (lumpectomy day)—*I plan to go into the operating room, gaining strength from Zephaniah 3:16, 17 as well as the first five verses of Psalm 103. Wally [my brother] came from Bend today to be with Mom. I hate it that—on top of everything else she has to cope with on a daily basis—she now has my cancer to worry about!*

February 5—*The surgeon feels certain he was able to remove all identifiable malignant tissue.*

February 6—*Went to see the surgeon. The pathology reports are not all back yet. No cancer showed up on the right breast ultrasound nor in the biopsied lymph nodes. That's good news. I have an appointment with a radiation oncologist. God, help me be strong for Jim and our sons!*

The first time I undressed for a shower, I had a bit of a shock. I hadn't thought that much about the form of my body being altered from the lumpectomy. For a moment I wondered if my new deformity merited the shedding of tears of not.

February 8—*I stayed home from church today and rested. Fell asleep very, very late. Awakened at the end of a dream in which I was coming down a walkway flanked by crowds on both sides while someone announced, "Look at her. She's battling cancer!" How bizarre—I can't escape my predicament even in sleep!*

February 9—*Got a phone call at 4:00 a.m. from Mom's assisted living residence. The nurse told me that Mom was on her way, via ambulance, to the ER with pain in her abdominal hernia. Jim and I jumped into our clothes and ran out to the car.*

In the ER we found Mom resting comfortably. She said her pain had subsided. How I hated seeing her there—I know she had to have felt frightened and alone when they transported her to the hospital.

The ER doctor released her two hours later with orders for a liquid diet the remainder of the day. We took Mom back to her apartment and tucked her into bed. She fell asleep right away. Jim took me home to rest before going to a program this evening at which I had the devotional. We left early and took Mom some liquids to "eat" and soft foods for tomorrow.

Before the meeting I visited with friends for the first time since they'd learned of my cancer. Their support and openly expressed affection felt good, though I had to present my body for hugs in such a way as to not have my surgery side bumped.

February 10*—Went to physical therapy to make sure the arm on my surgery side maintains its range of motion. I can't control cancer, yet I still have control over keeping my muscles flexible. I guess the best that I can do . . . is the best I can do.*

February 11*—The radiation therapist went over the pathology report with Jim and me. It was the first time we knew whether or not the biopsied sentinel node was negative or positive for cancer. It was negative. A BIG whew! The radiation oncologist also read from the pathologist's report that the margins around the excised lump were clean. Unfortunately, the tumor was 4.4 centimeters, rather than the 2-plus the surgeon had surmised from the ultrasound. I appreciate the fact that no one is forcing me to do what he or she thinks I should do.*

We rushed home from my appointment to pick up Mom and take her to her doctor's appointment to find the status of her abdominal hernia situation. After taking Mom back to her place, I felt deeply troubled. I just wanted to go home and cry (but as usual, there doesn't seem to be enough time). Life is so overwhelming.

Since I was still hurting from the surgery—and had Mom on my mind—I didn't feel very confident tonight during my 10-minute devotional at the ongoing seminar programs. My prescheduled topic tonight—either ironically or providentially—was entitled "Cope Through Hope."

"Do not fear. . . . The Lord your God is in your midst, the Mighty One, will save . . . He will quiet you with His love, he will rejoice over you with singing."
—Zephaniah 3:16, 17, NKJV

Scarred

The week following surgery I experienced shock every time I

disrobed to shower. When I first looked in the mirror at my scarred and misshapen chest (drain scar site, lymph node scar site, lumpectomy site), I tried not to cry. Yet I knew something that had been a part of my life for a long, long time was forever gone. I grieved quietly, though deeply.

During that time of private mourning, however, God drew me closer to His heart through a new mutually shared experience. He reminded me that He too had scars—in His hands, His feet, His side. What had been a part of His life for a long, long time would now forever be limited by the humanity He had chosen to assume—on my behalf.

His scars would forever bind to me to Him in a closeness that wouldn't have been possible had He not undergone the crucible that resulted in those scars for me.

I realized I no longer had to view my scars, and what was missing from my body, as losses. Rather I could embrace them as symbols. First, as symbols of victory.

Victory over a premature death, since the current cancer had been cut out.

Victory because the killer had been discovered and identified in ample time to do serious battle and perhaps ensure that I would enjoy extended life.

Second, I could embrace my scars as symbols of gratitude. Gratitude that my God was making good on His promise to be with me, personally, unto the end—whenever that end might come for me. Gratitude that He saw something in my flawed character worth refining through trial, pain, and uncertainty.

February 12—I took my first morning walk in a week. Though I was hurting some, the exercise surely felt good! I went to physical therapy, got my hair cut, and came home very tired.

Read in the newspaper that one can hire a male quartet to sing two love songs to a loved one on Valentine's Day. Wally and Victoria, along with Jim, think that would be a great surprise for Mom. She's had a very rough week.

Jim is learning to play the electric bass. What a guy!

February 13—No walk today. Saw my surgeon late morning. He re-

moved the stitches and went over the pathology report with us again. He too, like the radiation oncologist, expressed concern over the size of the tumor. For that reason he leans toward my undergoing chemotherapy. I'm beginning to wonder if treatment choices aren't a bit like Russian roulette.

February 14—Six years ago today Jim and I were in Frederick, Maryland, applying for a marriage license. Today we met a chemotherapy oncologist. But first we decided to step outside of painful reality and have a Valentine's date. We drove to Ashland and had a fabulous lunch in a little restaurant that has some great vegetarian dishes on its menu. How I am learning to cherish every moment I have with loved ones!

Next we went to a farmers' market and loaded up the cooler we'd brought along with fresh organic vegetables and fruits.

Spent almost two hours with the oncologist. She also feels that, because of the size of the tumor, I should undergo chemo (am I talking about me? I still have to pinch myself to realize this is really happening).

However, she said, "You have the data. It's your decision now. Go home and think about it. Pray, if you're a person of faith. And start keeping a diary. Maybe you could write a book someday about your experience with breast cancer that would encourage others."

That's one writing project I never intended to undertake—especially from a first-person perspective!

Mom raved about that male quartet that sang for her today at her residence. They even presented her with a long-stemmed red rose. I was so thankful we "kids" could do that for her since I had to be traveling or at medical appointments most of the day—instead of with her.

Mom had a beautiful little flower arrangement delivered to the house sometime today while we were gone. (Someone at her residence helped her order it since she can't see to read the phone book.) It's a beautiful arrangement of fresh-cut springlike flowers, and came with a tan teddy bear bearing the sweetest little expression on its face.

Always thinking of others

After retirement from 43 years of teaching, Mother still continued reaching out to others through homemade cards of encouragement, sympathy, and congratulations. However, when literally overnight she became blind from macular degeneration, she could no longer see to make cards. Even so, she could *feel* well enough to dress teddy bears and have them sent (along with an encouraging scripture) to people who needed comfort or support.

Jim and I were constantly packaging her newly dressed bears and running them to the post office. We called this Mom's special ministry, her burden bear ministry.

February 15—I helped with a special music at the Ashland church today, though I was pretty tired. Spent the afternoon with Mother, as I could tell she was not feeling well, physically or emotionally.

February 16—Mother didn't answer her phone this morning when I called her. I quickly phoned the front desk—receptionist said Mom had been vomiting.

Jim and I hurried over and immediately ordered an ambulance. All signs pointed to Mom's having a bowel blockage. X-rays at the hospital revealed that to be the case. Wally and Victoria drove over from Bend, about four hours away. Doctor couldn't operate today because of [the coumadin] Mom takes. She's having fresh frozen plasma intravenously all night plus vitamin K shots to thicken her blood.

I had a prayer with Mom before I left the hospital. She loves her night nurse and told me to dress a teddy bear and get it to her by tomorrow, as that is also the nurse's birthday. Mom could be on her deathbed (and maybe she is) and she'd still be thinking of others.

Am I scared for Mom? You'd better believe I am!

Dear God, it feels as if the sky is falling in!

February 17—This morning the surgeon told us confidentially, "My concern is that your mother won't make it through this operation because of her heart." We said goodbye to her, knowing that it might be our last farewell on this earth. Suddenly the value of the little bear Mom sent us on Valentine's Day skyrocketed.

Dear God, I thought, how much more can I take?

As we walked beside Mom's gurney toward the operating room Mom asked that I send a bear to Chaplain John, who facilitates her grief recovery group at her assisted living residence. John was having his hip replaced today. So I made myself a note to get one of Mom's bears for him, but spent the next three hours praying.

She survived the surgery and went to ICU! There is power in prayer! A wonderful ending to a long and exhausting day for all of us . . .

February 18—*Mom's signs were holding, and she was released to short-term care. My sister-in-law had to get back to Bend to work her nursing night shift. Wally stayed to be with Mom so Jim could take me to have my chemo portacath put in (yep, we're going with the chemo). That way the chemo meds will go into a much larger vein than the ones in my arms. The three of us went out to eat, and then I made a short presentation at the seminar again before returning to the hospital to be with Mom.*

February 19—*Had the chemo port surgically inserted after visiting Mom in the morning. Going to OR for the second time in three weeks was déjà vu.*

February 20—*Wally went to Mom's hospital in the a.m. so Jim and I could get some rest. About 11:30 a.m. we "took over" for the rest of the day. A nurse asked why I was so tired. I shared a bit about my cancer-related journey.*

"How are you even surviving?" she asked. I just shook my head and pointed heavenward. She nodded with understanding.

"What would we do without Him?" she smiled.

I responded, "We wouldn't. It's as simple as that."

I tried to lie down on the window seat of Mom's room in order to rest, but just couldn't seem to get comfortable. The surgically inserted portacath was giving me some pain. I got home about 7:00 p.m. Tomorrow I need to get Mom's bill paying caught up. There's been too much going on!

February 21—*When I got to the hospital this morning, I learned that Mom had fallen out of bed during the night. Yet she was doing well enough to be transferred to a nursing home that day. The rest of the day was taken up with my physical therapy appointment, Mom's transfer, and going back and forth to her residence to get clothes, etc., which she needed.*

Mom needed a lot of reassurance, since she was in a new place with new caregivers. They were all very reassuring, but the nursing home is very noisy, compared to her residence and the hospital. My heart constantly goes out to her because of her blindness. She is eating a bit more—mostly liquids. I got home about 8:30 p.m. and started returning phone calls.

Today I began reading Dr. Larry Burkett's book, Nothing to Fear—

The Key to Cancer Survival. *It's about faith, but is also filled with practical advice for what I'm going through.*

February 22—*Jim stayed with Mom this morning so I could rest. I went this afternoon. Mom was still on a liquid diet. She is listless, but not in much pain. Though my postsurgical pain is the strongest at night, I'm not thinking too much about my stuff. I'm very concerned about Mother, though!*

Sunday, February 23—*I began reading a book about a man—an M.D.—with cancer (though not my kind) who had surgery but opted not to have chemo. I keep wondering about my decision to have chemo before radiation. I keep praying that if it's not to God's liking, He'll block it.*

February 24—*Such dark news today! Via e-mail I learned that a friend of mine just died of leukemia. This weekend will also be the memorial service of a college classmate and friend. She just passed away—ovarian cancer.*

Mom ate only two spoonfuls of solid food today. Jim, who is such a great encourager, made even that possible. He is about as exhausted as I am. What a blessing from God is that man!

It breaks my heart to see Mother so feeble and listless. Yet—wouldn't you know it—she told me this evening, in a weak voice, to be sure to give one of her teddy bears to Viola, her roommate.

God's treatment plan

During these weeks of feeling so overwhelmed, the nightly sight of my healing scars in the bathroom mirror became reminders that Christ's scars represent a treatment plan He had from "the foundation of the world" (Ephesians 1:4; John 17:24) to fight the cancer of sin.

How I love Him for all the provisions He made on my behalf! Looking beyond the cancer, I could focus on this newfound, scar-shared closeness with my blessed Redeemer (Psalm 16:11).

Sure, I admit these changes of perspective didn't come overnight. Yet focusing on His scars instead of mine helped me stay sane during our personal chaos. After all, those unsightly jagged red lines that cost Him His life will prolong mine—and Mother's—forever.

REMINDER
We lean on God's heart by often thanking Him for His scars,
symbols of an eternal escape from the cancer of sin.

MEDITATION
*"Then He [Jesus] said to Thomas, 'Reach your finger here, and look at
My hands; and reach your hand here, and put it into My side. Do not be
unbelieving, but believing'" (John 20:27, NKJV).*

---

* In 2004 the Review and Herald Publishing Association published and released this
manuscript in book form under the title *Staying Vertical: A Spiritual Tool Kit for Christ-centered Living in an Out-of-balance World.*

Chapter 6

Preparing for the Inevitable

"I am telling you now before it happens,
so that when it does happen you will believe that I am He."
—Jesus[*]

hrough the years I've noticed that the world doesn't stop simply because *I* happen to be experiencing a crisis of gargantuan proportions.

Truckers still deliver stock to grocery stores. Kids still tease each other on their way to school. Birds still sit on telephone lines. Stoplights still turn red and green. Bills still arrive in the mail. Television anchors still share the world's news every 24 hours.

Yet in the days immediately following my cancer diagnosis, I was overwhelmed by . . . well, everyone else's apparent normalcy. I wanted to yell at the world, "OK, everybody, just *stop!* Stop what you're doing! How can you just go about your familiar daily routine when *I'm* so desperately trying to prepare for the crisis ahead?"

Perhaps this background of normalcy is precisely what makes personal trauma stand out in such bas-relief. Those facing imminent challenges struggle to be in a "state of readiness" while everyone around them just seems to just go with the flow.

Sometimes those of us facing sudden challenges don't even know how to fit the new demands of a crisis into our normal routine.

February 24, 2003*—At the doctor's office they said I might feel better during treatment (the balding part) if I had a couple of wigs to wear out in public. So I ran into a wig shop on the way home from today's first visit to Mom. Trying on wigs made my stomach tight. Even though my body* *already bears the marks of cancer treatment, I still feel as if this is happening to someone else.*

The gum-popping clerk at the wig shop kept referring to each wig as she: "Oh, she looks a lot better on your head than *she* does."

Only one wig in the shop even halfway worked, so I took *her* home. When I put *her* on, however, and looked in the mirror all I could do was shake my head and name *her* for what *she* looked like sitting atop my head: Hedgehog!

The following week the American Cancer Society furnished me with a free wig, which I also named for how she looked on my head: Muskrat.

In one last act of desperation, I visited another wig shop, where I acquired—The Silver Fox.

The original names of the wigs were Cappuccino Mist, Applause, and La Petite Jazz. As I renamed them, I felt like the Babylonian captors who couldn't relate to the original names of the three worthies, giving them instead other names to better reflect their new context: Shadrach, Meshach, and Abednego. Suddenly I was relating to fiery trials in a much different way than I'd ever done before.

I took the wigs to a beauty shop. A beautician, for a minimal fee, clipped them into similar styles and then cut my own hair to look as much like theirs as possible. I kept thinking, *This is ridiculous! I don't have time for this.* Yet I did need to sandwich in—between Mom's medical emergencies—my own personal preparation for the emotional, as well as the physical, changes about to transpire in my life. After all, one Bible writer pointed out that "a prudent person foresees the danger ahead and takes precautions" (Proverbs 22:3, NLT).

I supposed I should feel thankful that I'd at least been given fair warning. Yet I couldn't help wishing the apostle Paul had pronounced the same blessing over me that he pronounced over the centurion and Roman soldiers on the ship, that "not a hair will fall" (Acts 27:34, NKJV).

No, I thought, *I can't control my hair falling out. But I can have a little control over what I'll look like* after *it happens.* So I practiced learning how to shampoo and style Hedgehog, Muskrat, and The Silver

Fox. I took pictures of them in various "activities" and sent photos to my kids with such captions as "Here are Hedgehog and Muskrat taking their first swim together."

I made up jokes about being "all wigged out." At times I could get my family and friends to laugh, but my heart was filled with an unspeakable dread concerning the unknown.

February 25—Mother is eating somewhat better today. We spent quite a bit of time with her again. She's too tired to talk on the phone and didn't have a good time in physical therapy. She had me put together a get-well bear for her roommate, Viola. Jim and I had prayer with Mom and Viola before we left for tonight's seminar program.

My presentation at that ongoing seminar was all right but not excellent. I'm very tired.

"Plan ahead—
it wasn't raining
when Noah
built the ark."
—Bumper sticker

Couldn't fall asleep until sometime after 1:00 a.m. I had been reading some more about chemotherapy and am very apprehensive about this being the right decision. However, when I consider the alternative . . . I just don't know.

I'm concerned that I'm going into this too physically and emotionally depleted—because of the needs of my precious mother. God, please be with me! All I could do was lie in bed listening to Jim breathe and thanking God for him in my life at this juncture.

February 26—Mom is eating MUCH better today. She was proud of her breakfast intake. A friend spent the morning with her, and Mother appreciated that.

I had my chemo in-service today. The instructing nurse had me sit on one of the chairs in which I'll be having strong toxins transfused into my body. Along the corridor leading to the hospital's infusion center, I passed two bald women waiting in examination rooms. I remembered Hedgehog, Muskrat, and The Silver Fox sitting at home, up on the shelf in my closet. It still doesn't seem real.

The nurse gave me long lists of possible side effects from the chemo, as well as precautions I must take. For example, I won't be able to pet the cats for the next three and a half months because they might transmit some infection to my skin or respiratory system.

The nurse, in a cheery voice, did say I should continue my social life to keep my spirits up. However, she added, it would be a good idea if I wore a nose mask. (H'mm, that doesn't sound too social to me. "Hello, Carolyn! Glad you could join us for the birthday party. Would you like for us to hang up your sweater and nose mask, or would you like to continue wearing them?")

I remember that one of the patients receiving chemo that day was an upbeat great-grandmother. She told me that she had had a "pizza-haircutting" party for her great-grandchildren when her hair had started falling out. She had let the kids cut her hair and then shave her head. She concluded, "We all had a good time." More thoughtfully she added, "I've lost control over most of the things in my life right now. So I make sure I control what I can. That helps me cope emotionally."

The nurse told me I'd probably lose most of my hair within seven to 14 days following next Monday's initial treatment. I kept telling myself, "That's not going to be such a big deal."

Jim was by my side during this session and extremely supportive, as usual. *Dear God,* I silently prayed, *thank You for that man in my life! I don't deserve his love and kindness and good humor and faith.*

After the doctor's visit Jim said, "Enough of the heavy stuff. Let's turn the rest of today into a date. Woman, I'm taking you out to dinner!"

February 26 (continued)*—I'm compiling a three-ring binder that I've entitled Carolyn's Cancer Survival Kit. It will contain Bible promises I've been amassing, letters from well-wishers, and musical pieces I want to learn while I'm doing chemo and radiation.*

February 27*—Mom is not doing well again today. "She hardly ate anything," Jim said after his first of three trips over there today. I am so concerned about her and just wish I could lay hands on her and have all her medical problems go away. I just continue to pray for her—that whatever's suppose to happen . . . will.*

February 28*—I wasn't feeling too well this morning and am concerned about starting chemotherapy. I have a sore throat and am slightly chilled. I've been over to see Mom twice today, and Jim's been over there three times.*

Concerning another dark topic, it appears that our country is about to go to war in Iraq.

Although this week has been a challenging one, I'm glad the doctor's office is letting me know what to expect. That way I can prepare in advance and be as ready as possible.

Everyday reminders

I'm so glad that that no matter what cancer is eating away at our lives God still enables us to plan ahead every day.

On several occasions Jesus revealed future events so His disciples could prepare for them (see Matthew 24:25; John 13:19; 14:29).

However, along with dire prophecies, Christ also gave reassuring reminders. These reminders, which often accompanied Christ's unsettling predictions, hold true for us today. Most of us are still learning that "normalcy" just doesn't exist on Planet Earth . . . not for anyone! That's because the enemy of our souls is using every opportunity to maim (Job 2:7), deceive (Ephesians 6:11), and destroy (1 Peter 5:8).

Thank God that this world is not our final reality. What a loving Lord to remind us, in several domains, to plan ahead.

- "Watch and pray, that ye enter not into temptation" (Matthew 26:41).
- "Be always on the watch, and pray that you may be able to escape all that is about to happen, and that you may be able to stand before the Son of Man" (Luke 21:36, NIV).
- "Always be prepared to give an answer to everyone who asks you to give the reason for the hope that you have" (1 Peter 3:15, NIV).

Along with admonitions for readiness come reassurances that better times are on the way.

- "The word of God lives in you, and you have overcome the evil one" (1 John 2:14, NIV).
- "Be of good courage, and he shall strengthen your heart, all ye that hope in the Lord" (Psalm 31:24).
- "Fear not, little flock; for it is your Father's good pleasure to give you the kingdom" (Luke 12:32).

Personalizing a promise

May I share with you my own paraphrase of a favorite Bible warning-reassurance text? It's John 16:33. "In this abnormal world everyone experiences sin's cancer in one form or another. Yet, never lose heart! For I am about to effect . . . The Cure."

Dear friend, ask God to show you, even in the midst of your current struggles, one of His encouraging and sustaining truths. A truth that will enable you not only to plan ahead—get ready—for an eternity in heaven, but also help you hold on for today.

REMINDER
We lean on God's heart by heeding
His cautions and claiming His promises.

☙❧

MEDITATION
"Let us rejoice and be glad and give him glory! For the
wedding of the Lamb has come, and his bride has made herself ready"
(Revelation 19:7, NIV).

⋆ John 13:19, NIV.

Chapter 7

All Wigged Out!

"Instead of well-dressed hair, baldness . . ."
—Isaiah 3:24, NIV

As I approached the date of my first chemotherapy treatment, Mother's health continued to decline. And, come to think of it, I wasn't feeling so great either.

March 1, 2003—I'll not be going anywhere this weekend except to pop in on Mom. I must have caught this bug in the nursing home. It's so hot in there and it's so cold outside. I probably got overheated and then chilled. Lots of tightness in my chest and increasing sore throat. I suspect I've just worn myself out.

March 2—I didn't go visit Mom today because I didn't want to spread my bug. The last thing she needs now is a cold or the flu or walking pneumonia. Jim was there three times, though. What a gift from God that man is to all of us! Mom is having lots of back pain. Her lack of appetite makes us very concerned. I don't know where to put my worry "energy"—there's just so much going on!

God's timing

The following morning the telephone rang. Corleen Johnson, the women's ministries director of the Oregon Conference, was calling to ask if I would share a devotional at an upcoming prayer conference. She said that one of the presenters had had to cancel. I explained to her why I couldn't help her out.

"I hadn't heard of your cancer diagnosis!" she exclaimed. "In fact, I hadn't intended to call you today, except—except your name came up twice this morning in our departmental worship. I don't even remember why. That made us think that maybe God was impressing us to pray for you. But we didn't know why."

I listened in amazement as she spoke.

"Just a minute," she interrupted herself. "I'll call my assistant in here and turn on the speaker phone. Would you allow Diane and me to say a special prayer for you right now?"

I was moved beyond words at God's timing. Recently He had seemed somewhat distant. Yet suddenly this amazing phone call, and on one of my cancer journey's darkest days.

Tuesday, March 4—*Jim came in from the nursing home and said he's afraid we're losing Mom. We both decided I needed to go visit her—with my nose mask on. I did. We visited, and I had prayer with her. She thanked us as she always does.*

March 5—*This evening Federal Express brought some head coverings I had ordered from the American Cancer Society catalog . . . scarves and hats for when I lose my hair.*

March 6—*A wonderful young friend has agreed to spend some time each day with Mom when I can't be there. It will be a good match, and Mom will have company. Thank You, God!*

March 7—*I'm starting to have quasi-nightmares about losing my hair. Must be my subconscious working overtime.*

I'm adding another organic nutritional supplement to my immune system therapy. Feels good to do what I can—when so much is beyond my control.

Tonight—*when Jim was over at youth vespers—I sat down at the keyboard and started playing through an old hymnbook of Mother's. As I mentally sang the comforting words, tears started coming. I realized that during these past few weeks I haven't taken much time to cry—especially about what's happening to Mom. There just hasn't been much time, actually. Mom is slipping from our grasp. Jim is doing everything he can to support both of us, and he's exhausted too. The immediate future is so uncertain— for us, for our country.*

Dear God, help!

March 9—*Spent time with Mother, about four hours today. She is so sweet about everything, but she continues to fail. She tried to eat a little bit of food. All I can do is affirm, comfort, assist, and come home to cry.*

March 10—Stopped to see Mom this morning before Jim drove me to my first chemo treatment. I wept all the way to the hospital—for Mom, mostly, wondering how all this is going to play out. She's the most faithful, long-term, and closest friend I've ever had.

First treatment

Outside the hospital I squared my shoulders and walked in to that first chemo treatment as if I had a job to do. In fact, I'd dressed that morning as if I were going to a job that had an upscale dress code. I figured that fighting cancer was my current job. Therefore, I wanted to have a positive mental outlook and be ready for teamwork with the professionals caring for me.

In the infusion room a nurse hovered about while the doctor slipped in and out. I looked about the room and thought, *All these patients, including me, have chosen this extreme treatment in hopes of eradicating our cancers.*

Focusing on the Bible texts in my lap that I'd brought along to memorize, I couldn't help remembering the extreme measures to which heaven had gone in order to eventually eradicate the disease of sin on this planet.

I noticed that the other patients—men and women from their early 20s to early 70s—were all in various stages of hair loss. For me it would only be a matter of time. Indeed, cancer is no respecter of persons! Neither is sin and its baleful results.

March 23—I keep tugging at my hair to see if it's ready to fall out . . . but not yet. I've heard it can fall out anywhere between Day 3 after chemo and Day 21. The average time is 10 to 21 days after the treatment—but it's often on Day 14. I'm on Day 13. My scalp is itching and aching, perhaps from the power of suggestion?

March 24—Aha! Today's the day, I think. Every little brush of my hand through my graying mane was yielding one to five hairs. Then I washed it. When I'd finished blow-drying it, the hairbrush had collected enough hair to nest a small family of robins!

Why does it have to start falling out on such a cold, drizzly day?

I wondered. I fought back panic. I knew this would happen, I tried to reassure myself. Hedgehog, Muskrat, and The Silver Fox—my three musketeers—are waiting to be summoned into service. Everybody at the infusion center told me this would happen. The books all said it would happen. So why am I panicking? I guess . . . because it IS happening! Yikes!

Now I feel bad that I've complained about having problem hair all my life. And then about its turning from strawberry blond to silver. But when the rubber meets the road, I am belatedly thinking . . . hey, wait a minute! My hair isn't so bad after all!

The private panic

Incredulously I watched that morning as strands of my bangs did silent free falls into the sink. The knowledge that I'd be completely bald within a week seemed absolutely hideous!

***March 24 (continued)**—Just last night I was reading a book by a cancer survivor. She told about how her hair had started falling out when she was on an airplane. So she just got a can of hair spray and sprayed it all over her head. Her hair stayed on her scalp until she got home!*

I wanted to scream, to get out of my own body and away from any remaining cancer cells.

Where was my faith in God now?

How much do I trust? I wondered. There at the sink I knew I must grapple with two realities.

Dear God, I prayed, *here we go! Nothing in my life has prepared me for this—so I'm going to wrestle with You until You replace my panic with peace!*

And we went into a clinch. As God and I wrestled, two realities became very clear to me.

- Reality 1: I might not ever escape cancer this side of heaven, for this world is not my home (as that old gospel hymn affirms).
- Reality 2: No matter what is going on in my life, the joy of the Lord must *still*—and *always*—be my strength (as my chosen cancer journey theme text states).

In *The Ministry of Healing* author Ellen White states, "Nothing tends more to promote health of body and of soul than does a spirit of gratitude and praise. It is a positive duty to resist melancholy, discontented thoughts and feelings—as much a duty as it is to pray."[1]

I wrestled with God that horrific morning "to resist melancholy, discontented thoughts and feelings," and steeled myself against crying. Then a certain peace crept into my heart and calmed it.

March 24 (continued)—This isn't worth shedding tears over, I decided. I'm not the only person in the world to lose my hair. Besides, I've been telling everyone who brings up the subject that hair loss is the least of my worries. And it has been—until now!

How do You want me to deal with this, Lord? To put it all in perspective?

Suddenly I wondered if anyone had ever written a bluegrass song about chemotherapy. I met the urge to cry by quickly jotting down some words that came to mind. When I finished my set of lyrics, the urge to cry had passed. I entitled my totally impromptu composition "The Chemo Breakdown." Then pulling myself together, I answered Jim's breakfast summons.

Entering the kitchen, I held out a fistful of hair, smiled, and said to my husband (as nonchalantly as I could), "It's starting."

He rose to the occasion. "Ah, so then we'll be styling your hair with a wet washcloth?"

After grace I sang him my newly composed song over oatmeal, and we both laughed. He quipped about my composition going platinum at cancer treatment centers, hospices, and Race for the Cure rallies. Then we grew silent.

My eyes met his, and I saw that he was crying too.

> "Even with no hair, I can still 'worship the Lord in the beauty of holiness' (Psalm 29:2)—with His help, of course."
>
> —Journal entry

Comfort 101

Later that day I looked through a Bible concordance, trying to find an encouraging text. In Psalm 40:12 David likens the number of his iniquities to the number of hairs on his head. Wryly I thought, *If this is my case as well, I'll soon be perfect, given the amount of hair I'm losing!*

Fighting intermittent depression and panic, I put out the hair-loss word, via e-mail, to some of my closest supporters. Their responses soon filled up my e-mailbox.

A former student reminded me: "With or without hair, you'll still be everything you are now—church member and musician, wife, mom, friend, special daughter, and caregiver. None of these roles require hair!"

Another long-ago student pupil: "You've always been such a beautiful woman [is that why she was always an A student in my classes?], and I'm sure that losing your hair won't make any bit of difference. You'll just have fewer obstructions for letting your spirit shine through."

A former colleague encouraged, "You are a beautiful blond [I decided to keep *her* on my list of friends too!], and you'll be an even more beautiful *bald* because there's no dimming that light that shines from within! You're His girl, His beloved daughter."

A recent coworker observed, "Well, I suppose a little baldness between friends is a small price to pay, considering the alternative."

A longtime family friend responded, "Writing a song—what a great way to deal with the loss of hair. I can hardly wait to hear 'The Chemo Breakdown.'"

One former classmate (a musician) and his wife wrote, "Keep your chin up and remember . . . when in doubt . . . capo![2] Can't wait for the sequel. We're thinkin' of ya."

Another former classmate buoyed up my spirits with "Bless your heart, my friend. For standing up to it with a grin, and the willingness to write about it, you've my renewed respect."

My son Kent responded, "Mom, it's good you have a well-shaped head. I'm sorry that I'm not there to sweep up after you. [Ah, how sweet!] Let us know what you need, if anything (aside from a magic bottle of Cancer-Be-Gone or Hair-Be-Full). I hope that you are able to rest in Abba's arms."

Hair today, gone . . .

I looked out the window. Despite the drizzly day, my heart warmed to the encouragement God was sending me through some of

His own. Maybe losing one's hair wouldn't be such a big deal after all.

After pondering it, I realized that perhaps the only hair that's really worth looking at is the hair that's as "white like wool" and "white as snow" and frames the loving face of the One who paid the ultimate price for the cancer of sin (Revelation 1:14).

I was intrigued by the fourth verse of Isaiah 46. Read it with me.

> "Even to your old age, I am He,
> And even to your gray hairs, I will carry you!
> I have made, and I will bear;
> Even I will carry, and will deliver you" (NKJV).

What a beautiful promise that is!

Didn't He promise a long time ago that His Father has even numbered the hairs on our heads—whether the count is 40,000 or a measly four (Matthew 10:30)? That promise also means that He is aware of everything we are going through. In the midst of one of my darkest journeys, God was already giving me indications that He was aware of everything happening in my life.

After all, hadn't He orchestrated—with perfect timing—that unexpected phone call from Corleen and Diane, now two new prayer partners? One way or another, I was going to be OK. Nothing comes as a surprise to God—not even the loss of one's hair.

Five days later, when it was time, I went to the closet shelf on which my three wigs were perched. With a renewed sense that God was in control, I reached for—The Silver Fox.

REMINDER
We lean on God's heart by acknowledging His sovereignty over every event in our lives.

MEDITATION
"Are not two sparrows sold for a penny? Yet not one of them will fall to the ground apart from the will of your Father. And even the very hairs of

your head are all numbered. So don't be afraid;
you are worth more than many sparrows"
(Matthew 10:29-31, NIV).

---

[1] Ellen G. White, *The Ministry of Healing* (Mountain View, Calif.: Pacific Press Pub. Assn., 1905), p. 251.

[2] In other words, tighten the strings—and raise the pitch—of your guitar!

Chapter 8

Health to Thy Navel
and Marrow to Thy Bones

"O Lord, heal me, for my bones are troubled.
My soul also is greatly troubled."
—Psalm 6:2, 3, NKJV

Along time family friend saw the handwriting on the wall concerning Mother's state of health and my upcoming cancer
treatment. Her foresight prompted this sad bit of advice:
"Carolyn, I think you should start working on your mother's obit-
uary as well as on plans for a memorial service. You don't know
what lies ahead."

Though I felt terribly unfaithful to Mother doing so, I followed
the friend's advice.

*March 16, 2003—I finally got to go see Mom again since I'm feeling
stronger. I wheeled her outside for fresh air and sunshine, but we came in
soon, as she said it felt too cold to her.*

*I lay in bed tonight and faced the fact. Mother is dying. I asked God
how to pray, how to grieve, how to cope. So much around this house reminds me of the blessing we've had to have her so close to us these past
two years.*

Her eating bib.

*The little battery-operated high-density light to help her better see her
food because of the macular degeneration.*

Her favorite foods in the cupboard in anticipation of future meals with us.

Her electric easy chair.

Priscilla, the cat, that she so delights in holding on her lap.

All these shared experiences are over. I know it in my very soul, and it's breaking my heart!

I also remember those long and fatiguing days of helping Mom in her apartment, of shopping for her, of listening to her frustration over lost eyesight, of counting out her pills and vitamins into tiny containers, of paying her bills, of balancing her checkbook, of going home . . . and collapsing.

Then I remember Jim—bless his big, sweet heart—who would always say, "We won't always have Mom with us—let's just make her as happy and as comfortable as we can while we still have her. What more can I do to help you and her?"

How Jim's words and example have taught me what being like Jesus is all about!

New challenges

A parallel crisis—more serious than hair loss—had also developed the previous week. Mother, because of a serious kidney infection, had been rushed to the hospital yet again. As she improved, however, her doctor gave permission for her to return to the nursing home. I was so grateful that Wally, my brother, was coming again to spend time with her. That gave Jim and me some relief.

"If these bones ain't hurtin', it means they ain't movin'."

—Jim Sutton

We were all delighted when Mom told Wally that her back wasn't hurting anymore. I, on the other hand, was headed for a new experience with pain.

I'd never thought much about how bone marrow helps keep one strong and energetic. That is, not until the day my white blood count—following the first chemotherapy treatment—dropped down to 1.9.* Quickly my doctor ordered daily injections that would stimulate the bone marrow to produce more white blood cells.

Jim and I celebrated our sixth wedding anniversary by driving to the hospital for my Neupogen shots. The nurse administering the daily injections warned, "When this med takes effect in about four days, be prepared for some major pain."

Now, I've never desired pain. Yet, because of my compromised immune system, I found myself wishing the medication would start working—no matter how bad it might hurt.

March 19—Slept only about two hours. That skin irritation thing was really burning. I've been lying here thanking God for all the blessings in my life and how He's led me in the past and kept His hand over me. With Nehemiah, I too can say I owe everything to the "good hand of my God upon me" (Nehemiah 2:8).

March 20—Had sort of a blow today when I learned that my white count (instead of going up) had dropped from 1.9 to .7, which means at least two more of those shots—megadoses now. So I had one today and came home, trying not to be depressed.

The doctor wants to start me on an antibiotic since I'm a walking cipher ready to turn into whatever passing disease wants to take me out.

Three days after the first Neupogen injection, I began to feel a bit achy. *If this means my immune system is getting stronger and my marrow is making white blood cells again,* I thought, *bring on the pain!*

Little did I know!

The next morning I woke up with every joint in my body silently screaming. Yet I knew this pain meant that the bone marrow was at work making new, badly needed white blood cells.

A quick checkup call from my doctor's office gave me permission to take some light pain medication. What helped the most over the next few days of suffering was remembering that this pain was an indicator of something very positive. My immune system was being strengthened to resist infection—precisely *because* of this very painful bone marrow activity.

Again wisdom from the Scriptures brought spiritual insight to my physical challenges. Paul, in Hebrews 4:12, describes the Word of God as being powerful, sharp, and able to penetrate between the joints and marrow. It even discerns my thoughts and hidden motives. Now, *that* can hurt!

Yet, the resulting spiritual and even emotional pain, caused by spiritual conviction, is a very clear indicator of something most positive occurring at the level of the soul. The spiritual immune system is growing stronger precisely *because* the pain-inflicting sword of

God's Word is at work. On the other hand, I have no spiritual immune system without God in my life. I am incapable of fighting off the temptations and the disease of sin on my own.

The writer of Proverbs 3:7 and 8 reveals heaven's Neupogen shot to build the spiritual immune system back up. "Be not wise in thine own eyes: fear the Lord, and depart from evil," the writer says. "It shall be health to thy navel, and marrow to thy bones." Another rendition states that fearing God and shunning evil "will bring health to your body and nourishment to your bones" (NIV).

Fearing God and shunning evil are ways that we submit to God's will and lean on His heart for healing—however He chooses to work in the midst of our cancers. For only God can strengthen our spiritual immune system, and only when we give Him permission. Again, all I could do was cling to the One who had wrestled Jacob to the ground the darkest night of his life.

Holding on

During those days I thought a lot about Jacob. Like him, I knew that no one else could fight this battle for me.

Jacob was fully expecting his brother to wipe out his family the following day. Jacob already had enough to worry about without having a total stranger jump him in the middle of the night.

To make it worse, the Angel, during the midnight struggle, touched Jacob in a very sensitive place. The resulting pain crippled him.

I once heard a pastor say that sometimes—after we've had an encounter with God—we may limp for a while. Yet when we've been broken in different ways and at different levels, the broken places provide even more openings for God's grace to flow into our lives.

What about Jacob?

Jacob didn't understand why compounded tragedies had occurred in his life either. Yet at some point in his agony and struggle to survive, Jacob recognized Emmanuel, the God-with-us who has promised never to leave or forsake us (Hebrews 13:5).

In that moment Jacob recognized that God Himself had come to share his agony. So the exhausted, suffering patriarch simply held on—to God. He finally realized that throughout the long painful hours of that dark night he had been wrestling *in* the arms of God!

This realization encouraged Jacob to make a crucial decision. A decision just to give up and fall against the heart of God, submitting his terror and pain to the divine will.

With his last bit of energy, Jacob cried out, "I will not let You go unless You bless me!" (Genesis 32:26, NKJV).

In resounding affirmation to Jacob's request, God revealed the *promise* hidden in his *pain,* and brought him reassurance and hope (verses 24-32).

March 24—I know that three special women were praying for me yesterday, specifically about my bone pain. I think it was their prayers, along with Jacob's Angel, that helped me make it through one more crisis along this cancer journey.

Though today is dark and blustery, I once again commit my mother— and the rest of us—to the Sun of righteousness, who is shining in my heart. My residual pain this morning is nothing like it was yesterday. God is with me in this nightmare. I praise Him for His goodness!

What about you?

In your struggles, have you ever been crippled by physical or emotional pain you just couldn't understand? Have you done what Jacob did, simply relax in the loving arms of God?

REMINDER

We lean on God's heart by allowing Him to strengthen our spiritual immune system by wrestling with, and surrendering to, Him, within the safety and peace of His arms.

MEDITATION

"Ah, Sovereign Lord, you have made the heavens and the earth by your great power and outstretched arm. Nothing is too hard for you"
(Jeremiah 32:17, NIV).

⋆ Normal white blood count starts around 4.

Part II

At the End of the Rope

"The eternal God is your refuge,
and underneath are the everlasting arms."
—*Deuteronomy 33:27, NIV*

I used to do a lot of rappelling into caves.

Before going down a rope into a dark cave, however, we cavers always checked the condition of our ropes. After all, the rope was our guarantee of a safe arrival at the bottom of a vertical shaft. It was our assurance for getting back up out of the cave as well.

Once, when I had partially descended into a California cave known as Dragon's Breath, I saw—in the beam of my headlamp—that the rope a few yards below me had become tangled. Evidently the lower end of the rope had hit the irregular sides of the crooked shaft and knotted itself. Before I could descend to the base of the shaft I had to untangle the rope.

Fortunately I spotted, just below me, a formation shaped a bit like a saddle. I was able to lower myself enough to straddle this projectile, tie myself in, pull up the rope, and untangle it. I completed my descent.

Another aspect of rappel ropes, which we also checked before descending into a pit, was the *length* of our rope versus the *depth* of the pit into which we were about to rappel.

During my most active caving years I read everything about caves that I could get my hands on. Among the most terrifying caving stories I read was one about a man who went solo caving. He first checked the condition of his rope and found it to be strong.

However, he neglected to verify that the length of his rope was longer than the depth of the entry shaft of the cave he planned to explore. He naively began his rappel, came to the end of his rope 40 feet above the cavern floor—and fell to his death.

Sometimes life's dark surprises have unexpectedly "shortened" my "rope." As a result, I've felt as if I'd come to the end without enough emotional or spiritual footage to see me through the crisis.

I have felt, at times, that if God would only give me one—just *one*—"Because" answer to a "Why?" question, I could cling to my rope just a little bit longer.

In Part I, however, I shared that during my journey through cancer God did *not* give me any straight-on "Because" answers. Yet He *did* provide insights concerning how to hold on to my rope just a little bit longer.

More than just wanting me to cling to the end of my rope, God wanted me to learn how to *lean* on heaven's rope. Rather than giving me answers, God quietly showed me simple ways to lean more heavily on His heart—especially in times of personal crisis. Let's recap these ways.

- We lean on God's heart when we sit securely on the three-legged spiritual stool He has provided us: (1) His omniscience; (2) the encouraging examples of other survivors; and (3) His accessibility through our prayers.
- We lean on God's heart when we allow life's storms to be stepping-stones toward increased faith.
- We lean on God's heart when we trust Him with today—no matter now bleak tomorrow looks.
- We lean on God's heart by remembering that He wants us to have healthy souls even more than He wants us to have healthy bodies.
- We lean on God's heart by often thanking Him for His scars—symbols of our eventual and eternal escape from sin's cancer.
- We lean on God's heart by heeding His cautions and claiming His promises.
- We lean on God's heart by acknowledging His sovereignty over every event in our lives.

- We lean on God's heart by allowing Him to strengthen our spiritual immune system.

Yet what are we to do when tough stuff forces us to the end of our ropes, and the leaning option no longer seems feasible?

How I resonate with these words of C. S. Lewis: "You never know how much you really believe anything until its truth or falsehood becomes a matter of life and death to you. It is easy to say you believe a rope to be strong and sound as long as you are merely using it to cord a box. But suppose you had to hang by that rope over a precipice. Wouldn't you then first discover how much you really trusted it?"[*]

---

[*] C. S. Lewis, *A Grief Observed* (San Francisco: Harper, 1996), pp. 22, 23.

Chapter 9

Write It on My Heart

"Life is like an onion:
You peel it off one layer at a time, and sometimes you weep."
—Carl Sandburg

Physically and emotionally exhausted, Jim was the next family member to fall sick. A bad flu was making the rounds that spring.

His illness meant that he couldn't visit Mother at the nursing home. She didn't need exposure to any more germs. So, putting on my wig and nose mask and fighting the chemo-related fatigue, I began visiting her as frequently as I could.

March 17, 2003—I slept upstairs last night so Jim wouldn't have to keep stifling his cough for fear he'd contaminate me. I just couldn't sleep. I read. I prayed. I mourned for Mother's decline. For a long time I listened to Jim downstairs repeatedly clearing his throat and coughing. I felt so sorry for him.

I have a blood draw today to see what my red count is doing. I've had a good two-mile walk with my neighbor these past two days. Walking has felt good, but it tires me now. I have physical therapy this afternoon—don't want lymphedema to set in on my surgery side if it doesn't have to.

What's heaviest on my heart, though, is Mom . . . my mommy . . . my precious mother.

March 18—Visited Mom around noon. She seems to be rallying again! I'm glad, but what a roller coaster ride for her. She has also eaten much better today.

I took some of the letters she'd written to her mother years ago and read them to her. She seemed very interested in them, and we had a few chuckles.

Mother has written much about her family memories. She even dictated some of her recollections and experiences to Dad after becoming blind—so she wouldn't forget.

As I was reading to Mother, I suddenly realized that she's written enough to possibly incorporate into my current writing project. (Yes, another former project set on a back burner in order to deal with family medical needs. However, since I have no idea what mental and emotional shape I'll be in after completing cancer treatment, I've decided to put the pedal to the metal and churn out this manuscript before my second chemo treatment.) It's a book manuscript about how to individualize journal-keeping.[1]

So I asked Mom if she'd like to collaborate on this book manuscript. She said, "I'd love to. But how I could I collaborate with you, being blind and flat on my back most of the time?"

"Just do what you do when I bring you my speeches to critique," I told her. "I'll incorporate your writing into the existing manuscript after you've orally critiqued it. Then I'll read it out loud to you, and you can give your final input to the chapters."

"That sounds like a good plan," she smiled weakly.

Writing Mom on my heart

Each day as I took the newly revised chapter drafts to Mother's bedside, I'd pretend we were going to go on like this forever. I tried ignoring what I already knew—that my beloved mother was running out of time. Equally, I tried not to dwell on the thought that I too might be running out of time.

Mother would listen with interest as I read, and then give her input, slowly and in a weak voice.

Soon Mom could tolerate my reading only half a chapter at one sitting. She'd tell me, "I need to rest my mind a bit now. Could we finish reading that tomorrow?"

Toward the end we did well to get through even one paragraph an hour. As we neared the end of the manuscript Mother could concentrate on only two or three sentences before stopping to take a little break.

Her extreme weakness reminded me of one of my favorite literary characters, Beth in Louisa May Alcott's *Little Women*. As the young Beth was nearing death, yet still trying to sew, she would comment to her sisters that the needle was growing too heavy to hold. I'd always thought Ms. Alcott's depiction of Beth's predeath weakness was melodramatic. Now I knew better.

Because of my compromised immune system, an oncology nurse had advised me not to visit schools or nursing homes. Yet with Jim so sick, I couldn't bear to leave Mother without a family visitor each day. Just one of us dropping by meant so much to her.

Often I had strength for just one visit a day. Yet ever uppermost in my mind was the reality that our precious moments together were dwindling.

"One watches the elderly like you watch an infant— with an unflagging and unceasing vigilance."

—Kent Nerburn [2]

In a sense I suppose I wanted to be like Mary in the Bible. When time was running out for Jesus, Mary and Martha had the same opportunity to be with Him. Mary chose to spend every possible moment with Him in order to glean what she would need after Christ was gone. Her anointing His feet demonstrates her grip on the reality of His quickly approaching death. Martha, on the other hand, was still caught up in the mundane.

March 23—Jim is over the contagious part of his bug now, so he's again visiting Mom several times a day. She gently refuses food quite consistently now. Jim sits by her side and holds her hand. That seems to comfort her.

On days when I was too weak to visit Mother, we would talk on the phone as Jim held the receiver to Mother's ear. When my Neupogen shots elevated my white blood count enough, I would once again put on a face mask and drive myself back to the nursing home to be with Mom.

March 28—Spent more time with Mom today, but she just doesn't express interest in eating anything. She slowly sips various drinks, but even forgets when she is holding them. I talked about her part of the dedication for our book. She couldn't come up with a decision. I'll try again tomorrow.

Guess I've been overdoing it these past few days. I went to bed early while Jim went back over to visit with Mom.

The amount of hair I lost today was ridiculous. At the end of my shampoo in the shower there was a huge, wet, dark pile in the corner—all my hair. My hair has always been so thick that I could never even see my scalp. Now, wherever it parts, there's a one-inch-wide swath of pink scalp. I keep asking Jim if he'll help me shave my head, but he keeps saying, "Let's wait a little bit longer."

I suspect he's not any more anxious to see me totally bald than I am!

At least we had sunshine today—we needed that for a variety of reasons. Thank You, God!

March 31*—I took Mom's and my "Write It on Your Heart" manuscript—finally finished—to the post office today. I can't believe anything written under such ominous circumstances—by a cancer patient wearing a nose mask and her blind mother (who sometimes forgets she's holding a glass of water)—would have enough merit to be published. However, Mom and I did pray over our project when we first started it. The collaboration has given us hours of purposeful communication and also helped Mother recall and relive warm, fulfilling chapters in her own life.*

When I told Mom I'd sent in the manuscript, she sighed contentedly and emitted a weak "Oh, good! We finally wrote *a book together. I've wanted to do that for years!"*

April 1*—I awoke at 5:00 a.m. with a strong impression to pray for my mother. I hadn't felt an intensity like that since three days before my dad's death, when the same impression constrained me to do the same for him. I spent the next three hours in prayer before an open Bible—praying God's Word back to Him on behalf of my mother and her eternal destiny.*

I went to see Mother in the morning and was shocked by the change I saw—labored breathing despite an oxygen machine now. Her IV tubes had been pulled because they had begun aggravating her congestive heart failure and fluid-filled lungs. Her color was not good; her skin was drawn and starting to crack.

I quietly greeted her, and she mumbled, "Not a good day!"

"What's wrong, Mom?" I asked.

"Everything!" she responded.

"I'm going to find the nurse," I assured her.

She nodded.

Privately the nurse explained that malnutrition was breaking down Mom's organs, including her skin.

I fought tears behind my nose mask. Noticing, the nurse hugged me and told me how sorry she was.

I phoned Wally and told him what was happening. He said they'd be on their way. I went back to Mother's side and silently prayed for emotional control.

I don't know why I even asked Mom if she wanted me to read any e-mails to her that people had sent [that was her way of "writing" and keeping up with her friends]. She just shook her head.

All I could do was hold her—as best I could— through the guardrails and repeat the words of comfort, hope, courage, and assurance that God's arms were around her too. The Bible promises I'd read earlier that day came through my lips.

I felt Mom relax. For hours I stroked her hands and head and silently prayed. Caregivers changed her position from time to time. She sipped a bit of water, but said it came back up.

I dabbed moisturizing ointment on her lips. I told her I was so sorry she was uncomfortable. Only God knows how badly I wanted to cry out, "Mom, please don't go!"

Instead I asked Him to keep my voice steady. I reminded her how much I loved her. How much she was loved by family members and her former students. I spoke of the difference she'd made in the lives of so many people— and of a better time to come when Jesus would make all things new. I don't know how much she heard or understood.

Then, as was our habit, I said a little prayer with her (if I ever forgot and prepared to leave, she would always remind me to "pray with me"). After "Amen," I said, "I love you, Mom. I love you."

She rallied enough to murmur, "I love you too."

When it was time for me to leave for my Neupogen injection at the hospital, Mom had drifted into unconsciousness. Out in the car I sobbed like a baby.

Though exhausted from not enough rest the previous week because of Mother's ongoing crisis, I returned to the nursing home after my shot.

Jim came to relieve me. He stayed with Mother until Wally and Victoria arrived.

The end

My second chemotherapy treatment had been scheduled for the following morning. Jim and I stopped briefly by the nursing home on our way to the hospital in Medford. Mom's labored to breathe. She had remained comatose since the previous evening.

Leaving Mother in that little room—even with family members by her side—was one of the hardest things I've ever done!

April 2—Halfway through my chemo treatment Jim walked into the in-fusion room, blinking back tears. I could tell he was strug-gling to act normal.

I said, "You got a phone call, didn't you." He nod-ded and started crying. "She's gone," he said. "Wally just called. Mom is gone."

"My eye wastes away with grief."
—Psalm 31:9, NKJV

Careful not to bump the tube conducting the chemo drugs through my shoulder portacath, Jim leaned over and held me.

Mother had fought a good fight. The news of my cancer had taken its toll on her. So had a sudden bowel obstruction necessitating emergency surgery a few weeks earlier. Now it was all over. She was at rest.

I remember Mother saying to me one evening a few weeks earlier as we left her assisted living apartment, "Don't worry tonight. I'll drop off to sleep counting my blessings."

I like to think that's how she went to sleep in Jesus—counting her blessings.

The process

Cancer survivor Amy Givler states that grief is a process.[3] I wondered how long, in my particular grieving process, I'd be feeling this kind of pain.

In his book *Calm Surrender* Kent Nerburn makes this revealing statement about the death of a loved one. "When they [funeral preachers] have finished with their words, the dark truth still remains, and we can do no more than bow our heads before the mystery, and sit in silent grief until the balm of time reduces our pain to a burden we can bear."[4]

The pain of cancer was huge. Yet the pain of losing Mom was indescribable. I asked God to help me bear yet another loss, just two short years after the loss of my father.

I also began to wonder if the emotional strain I'd been under for the past few years (because of my parents' health problems) had negatively affected my body's ability to fight the onset of cancer. After all, Proverbs 18:14 warns, "The spirit of a man will sustain him in sickness, but who can bear a broken spirit?" (NKJV).

Though I was definitely broken in spirit, my first concern at this point was to get through the post-death necessities: obtaining death certificates, notifying family friends and insurance companies, sending obituaries to newspapers, planning Mother's memorial service.

"And God shall wipe away all tears."

—Underlined verse in my late father's Bible

We planned the date of Mother's memorial service around two considerations: when family members could conveniently arrive in town to attend, and when my post-chemo treatment white blood count would most likely permit *me* to attend.

Daily I prayed that I could emotionally survive this latest loss in my compromised physical condition. Knowing that pressing through tough times might somehow help me become a better person brought me a small measure of comfort.

I recalled Ellen White once writing, "Faith, patience, forbearance, heavenly-mindedness, [and] trust in your wise, heavenly Father are the perfect blossoms which mature amidst clouds and disappointments and bereavements."[5]

In the days immediately following Mother's death I also took a measure of comfort in the Resurrection. How true that "His [Christ's] resurrection . . . declares to all bereaved souls that 'them also which sleep in Jesus will God bring with him' [1 Thessalonians 4:14], and therefore the light of His resurrection falls in radiant beauty upon the graves where rest the dust of the holy dead."[6]

Though no one could ever take the place of Mother in my life, I hoped that eventually new friends and life experiences would also help me process the grief and bring a new kind of comfort.

I recalled how the biblical Rebekah, Isaac's beautiful young wife, comforted him after the death of his mother, Sarah (Genesis 24:67). No, Isaac didn't forget Sarah. In fact, he kept her tent erected—as a partial tribute to her—and into this tent he brought his new bride. Sharing warm memories of past closeness with his mother as well as longtime family traditions brought richness into this new chapter of Isaac's life.

When Isaac brought Rebekah into his mother's tent, the Bible says, "Isaac was comforted after his mother's death."

I too attempted to surround myself with warm memories and reminders of *our* family traditions. In a corner of my upstairs office I set out even more photographs and mementos of Mother's—beside Dad's now—in a little makeshift shrine. I grieved deeply and then waited to see how God would comfort me.

REMINDER
We lean on God's heart by honestly
grieving our losses before Him.

MEDITATION
"How long wilt thou forget me, O Lord? for ever? . . . How long shall I take counsel in my soul, having sorrow in my heart daily? . . . Consider and hear me, O Lord my God: lighten mine eyes, lest I sleep the sleep of death. . . . But I have trusted in thy mercy; my heart shall rejoice in thy salvation. I will sing unto the Lord, . . . because he hath dealt bountifully with me" (Psalm 13:1-6).

---

[1] Subsequently published in 2004, and released in book form by the Review and Herald Publishing Association under the title *Write It on Your Heart: How to Make Journaling Work for You.*

[2] Kent Nerburn, *Calm Surrender* (Novato, Calif.: New World Library, 2000), p. 66.

[3] Amy Givler, *Hope in the Face of Cancer,* p. 35.
[4] Nerburn, p. 98.
[5] Ellen G. White letter 1, 1883.
[6] Mike Mason, *The Gospel According to Job,* p. 384.

Chapter 10

Chemo Breakdown

"You have great physical ability and an iron constitution."
—An ironic fortune inside my Chinese fortune cookie
just after I was diagnosed with cancer

S truggling with grief—and against fatigue—I worked hard the rest of that week, taking care of the business of death. I notified family friends and insurance companies of Mother's passing and sent obituaries to newspapers in places she had lived.

We specifically scheduled Mother's memorial service to coincide with my new set of Neupogen injections boosting my white blood count. That way I could attend the service with a less-compromised immune system.*

The *real* "chemo breakdown"

Three days before my mother's scheduled memorial service, Jim found me on our bedroom floor at 4:00 in the morning. I was in pain and shaking violently. He drove me to the hospital for a blood draw.

Once there, he helped me ease into a wheelchair. My stomach felt queasy. My bones ached. As Jim pushed my wheelchair over the cracks between the marble tiles in the hospital floor, jarring pain shot throughout my body at the small bump of each crack.

The blood draw results revealed that my white count had just about bottomed out.

Though we didn't know it then, I was experiencing the statistical misfortune of being one in 5,000 to 10,000 whose body reacts to accumulated chemo drugs by going into shock because of near total loss of white blood cells.

Infusion nurses quickly notified my doctor in Medford. Diagnosing me as having neutropenic fever, she ordered me to the hospital in Medford, 25 miles away. I shivered under a pile of blankets in the back seat as my frightened and praying husband sped the car onto the interstate.

An hour later Jim watched silently from a chair in the corner of my isolation room in a Medford hospital oncology unit. Masked and gowned medical personnel scurried about my bed. One hooked up an IV to the portacath in my chest. Another attached tubing to a vein in my wrist. Someone else piled warm blankets atop my chilled body. A never-ending procession of individuals with clipboards entered the room, asked me questions, made notes, and left.

Every few minutes yet another medical technician would approach, pull back the bedding from somewhere on my body, and take vital signs or readjust a tube. Each time this happened a rush of icy air encircled me, reactivating my severe chill.

At first I felt embarrassed by strangers of both genders pulling aside my hospital gown to check on the various tubes. Wryly I remembered my own very modest mother—just a few weeks earlier—undergoing the same experience in the nearby Grants Pass hospital. One evening a male CNA walked into her room and asked, "May I take a look at your incision, Mrs. Roth?"

She responded wryly, "Why not? Everybody *else* is!"

I almost chuckled. It would be interesting to compare notes with her. Then I remembered . . . she was gone.

Out of control

Jim looked pale and drawn. I knew he needed to do things at home in preparation for family members who would soon arrive for Mother's memorial service. I told him to go on home and get a good night's sleep. I almost asked him to phone Mother when he got home, to reassure her that I was in good medical hands for the night. Then I remembered—again.

Why does my mind keep doing that? I numbly wondered as a nurse clamped a device on my finger in order to measure the percentage of oxygen in my blood. *And why is the pain so fresh every time I remember?* More and more, my life and my head weren't making a whole lot of sense.

That first night in the hospital I determined to stay as much in control of my situation as I could. *At least I can have my evening devotional,* I thought. From off of the bedside stand and onto my pillow I nudged my little pink Bible, a small notebook, and a red marker that I'd hastily dropped into the bag that I'd quickly packed for the hospital.

I was shaking too badly to write anything in my journal, so I simply turned to Isaiah 66:13, a verse I'd been frequently rereading since Mother's death. "As one whom his mother comforteth, so I will comfort you; and ye shall be comforted." How I craved that promised comfort!

> "My times are in thy hand."
> —*Psalm 31:15*

My chilled fingers next paged to 2 Corinthians 4. Before chemotherapy began, I'd made up a little laminated card containing verses 6-12 and 16-18. Memorizing them was my project during chemo treatments. Tonight the words swam together, yet some phrases stood out more than others: "perplexed, but not in despair"; "cast down, but not destroyed"; "though our outward man perish."

My room was next to the bustling nurses' station. That night, after checking my vital signs, a nurse placed the television controls in my hand and switched on the TV mounted overhead.

I really didn't care to watch anything. Yet feeling awash in loneliness, I desired some sort of company. Hoping that white noise in the background would help me drop off to sleep, I selected a TV shopping network and turned the volume down low.

Throughout the night I slept fitfully as the caregivers came and went. All I remember is hurting, feeling very cold, and trying not to get tangled up in all the tubing attached to my body.

Morning arrived and so did Jim, looking more haggard than ever. He and the doctor, one on either side of my bed, discussed my prognosis as if I weren't there. Jim happened to glance down at the little journal on the bedside table.

"What's this?" he asked me.

"It's a journal I brought to the hospital," I murmured. "But I didn't write anything in it."

"Well, somebody sure did," he countered. "The writing is with this red marker here, and it's in *your* handwriting."

"Really?" I asked. "What does it say?"

"Well, it looks like the 800 number for a TV shopping network followed by a long list of items to purchase. You must have scribbled all this during the night when your fever peaked."

"I don't remember writing anything down," I weakly protested.

"That's OK, darlin'," Jim said. "Yet with this telephone so handy and this long list of items to purchase, I'm just thankful I didn't leave the *credit card* with you!"

Getting colder

The first two nights I requested so many heated blankets that the weight of them on my body grew nearly intolerable. Finally I asked Darrell, a strapping thirtysomething nurse, if he could prop the door open. I'd heard it was warmer in the hallway than in my room. He said he would check with the doctor, since I was in isolation.

Soon he returned saying he could prop it open for short intervals—just long enough to take the chill out of my room.

With the door open, my room didn't feel so much like a morgue anymore.

"It's a whole lot warmer with the door open," I said gratefully.

Because of my weakness and multiple IV tubes, the nurses wouldn't allow me to get out of bed by myself. Because of increasing nausea, I needed to call for them more and more frequently.

Near midnight that second night, Darrell helped me back into bed and then asked, "How are you doing? I mean, *really* doing?"

I answered honestly, "I don't know. All I know right now is that my times are in His hands."

"You're absolutely right," Darrell agreed. "Only God knows what lies ahead. David wrote that all our days are numbered, even before we were born—with cancer or without. So it's all right, Carolyn, just to want His will to be done."

"Darrell," I began, "in this unit, is there very much—"

"Death?" he finished my question for me, as if used to discussing this topic.

I nodded, feeling the stubble from my recently shaved head catching on the inside of the cotton cap as it moved against the pillow.

"Yes, Carolyn," he answered quietly, "there's a lot of death here. You know, someday my wife and I want to be missionaries in a developing country. But for right now, this is my mission field. And it's a hard field to work. I grow to love my oncology patients. Then, all too often, I come to work only to find their beds empty. I just have to go into the linen closet and pull myself together before I can get on with my day."

"I'm sorry," I said, realizing anew how precarious my situation must be.

"By the way," he added, "I pray for my patients."

"Thanks, Darrell," I murmured.

As with most people, I had lived with a healthy fear of death. Yet Darrell had just told me that it's "all right" for God's will to be done—even if His will included my death at this point in my life.

I didn't know *what* to think anymore. What I did know had shrunk to a few miserable facts: 1. I knew that my cancer diagnosis had interrupted Jim's life and mine—perhaps forever. 2. I remembered, for once, that I couldn't telephone my mother for encouragement anymore because she was . . . dead. 3. I knew that family and friends were flying or driving to southern Oregon for her memorial service only two days away. 4. Finally, I knew I was too sick and weak to get myself even from the bed to the bathroom.

Warmth and light filtered through doorway where, with my doctor's permission, Darrell had propped open the door. How I wished I had the strength just to get up and walk through that doorway into the light and warmth.

"It's a whole lot warmer with the door open," I'd told Darrell, and suddenly I wondered if the glow through another doorway—offering relief from the coldness of life—might not also be drawing me. The door to death.

Maybe I had finally lost my fear of dying. Or was it that I just wanted a quick way out from all the pain?

REMINDER
We lean on God's heart when we allow
compassionate people to support and comfort us.

✺

MEDITATION
"Lord, remind me how brief my time on earth will be. Remind me that my days are numbered, and that my life is fleeing away. . . . An entire lifetime is just a moment to you; human existence is but a breath. . . . Hear my prayer, O Lord! . . . Don't ignore my tears. For I am your guest—a traveler passing through, as my ancestors were before me. Spare me so I can smile again before I am gone and exist no more"
(Psalm 39:4-13, NLT).

★ From this point on in my narrative, you will run across very few journal excerpts because the ensuing medical crisis stopped me from journaling altogether for a period of time.

Chapter 11

Room 2327, Bed A,
Patient 5296459-0 58Y

"The Lord is righteous in all His ways, gracious in all His works.
The Lord is near to all who call upon Him, to all who call upon Him in truth.
He will fulfill the desire of those who fear Him;
He also will hear their cry and save them."
—Psalm 145:17-19, NKJV

During my first two days in the hospital the only allowed visitor was Jim—after he'd scrubbed at the sink and masked up, of course.

I so longed for him to hold me! Yet he was permitted only to pat my feet through the pile of warmed blankets with his rubber-gloved hands. Touching me—even with gloved hands—would have risked additional infection.

Jim's drawn face, drooping shoulders, and uncharacteristically red eyes spoke of exhaustion. How faithfully he had cared for Mother's needs and supported my supporting her.

Now a host of family members and friends were descending on him for Mother's memorial service. The feeding and entertaining of these guests would fall squarely on his able, but weary, shoulders.

Despite augmented Neupogen injections, heavy antibiotics, and blood transfusions, my counts continued to drop. Mouth sores and skin rashes now added to my physical discomfort. Occasionally a hospital volunteer would appear at my doorway with a lovely flower arrangement someone had sent me, only to be turned away by a vigilant nurse. "You can't go in here," the nurse would say. "This is an isolation room. The fresh flowers might contain bacteria, and we can't take the risk."

The volunteer would then open the accompanying card and call out the message and name of the thoughtful party who had ordered the flowers.

Despite medication, one side effect from the chemotherapy continued to be pain. However, I prided myself on putting forth a gargantuan effort to appear cheerful, normal, and "together" when people entered the room. Yet my husband tells me I often came across anything but.

Early one morning, masked and gloved, Jim entered the hospital room. He recalls that the ensuing conversation with me went like this.

> "Don't take life too seriously, because you probably won't get out of it alive."
>
> —Anonymous quote on an e-mail forward

Jim: "Good morning, my darlin'. How are you feeling today?"

Me (weakly): "A little better, I think. In fact, I've been quite busy this morning."

Jim (looking at me under the pile of heated blankets): "Busy? Doing what?"

Me (pointing to the pitcher of water on the bedside stand): "I've been busy putting together this lovely flower arrangement."

Jim (taken aback): "Oh? And what kind of flowers have you been using in your arrangement?"

Me: "Well, can't you see? It's an artichoke bouquet!"

Jim (trying not to laugh at—or offend—my obvious sincerity): "Oh, sweetheart . . . [at a loss for words], how . . . *nice!*"

More visitors, sympathetic and otherwise

Though she was sympathetic to my mother's upcoming memorial service my oncologist decided that attending it would be too much of a health risk for me. In my heart I knew she was right. Though I remained stoic, she sensed my disappointment and let up a bit on the stringent no-visitors restriction. This permitted me to see family members who had traveled long distances to support us during this time of bereavement.

My heart broke for son Kent and his wife having to see their hospitalized mother—bald, pale, and emaciated. Moreover, embarrassing bouts of my nausea punctuated my brief visit with them.

Later when Aunt Evy, Mother's only surviving sibling, walked into the room with Jim and another close family friend, I fought hard not to cry. For with my aunt came a lifetime of family memories.

While talking with even my most empathetic visitors, I still sensed the truth of the following statement: "Anyone who has wrestled with serious illness in a hospital room, or received visitors there, will know that between the sick and the well, between the paralyzed life of the sufferer and the full, energetic outer world of the visitor, there exists a vast and nearly uncrossable chasm."[1]

As I visited with my aunt an unmasked cleaning woman entered my room and began sweeping around the edges of this sacred moment. When I murmured to my aunt, "Mom is gone," the janitor—a total stranger—exclaimed from the corner of the room, "She *is?*"

Quickly she rushed to my bedside. Her head intercepting my line of vision with Aunt Evy, she bent over me, firing a round of questions.

"When? How did it happen? Did you just find out *today?* Oh, I am *sooo* sorry! What are you gonna *do?* And here you are in the *hospital,* of all places!"

I sensed the woman was probably sincere. On the other hand, this exploding inquisition into the sanctity of my heart, already overflowing with grief and longing, nearly pushed me to the edge.

Uncharacteristically I wanted to yell at her, "Get out of my face! Don't make me share this loss one more time!"

Not trusting my emotions, I simply looked at Jim and said, "Could I please speak to you a moment . . . *alone?*" All others, including the well-meaning stranger, dutifully left the room. Then I broke down.

A moment later I called for my visitors and apologized for my abrupt request.

The above incident illustrates that one of grief's heaviest burdens is the reality that the sufferer must walk the valley alone. Other people often don't understand because they're not walking in the shoes of bereavement.

To the sufferer, on the other hand, others may seem callous—because life is going on, as usual, for *them*. Sometimes, however, others *are* callous.

Two mornings after my father's death the phone rang in my parents' home. I answered. A member of a local civic organization asked to speak with my father.

"That's not possible," I said quietly. "He passed away two days ago."

I assumed the man would mumble an embarrassed condolence and then terminate the conversation.

Instead he said, "Oh! Well—is *Mrs.* Roth there then?"

"No," I answered. "She's not."

"Well, then," said the man, irritation creeping into his voice, "isn't there *somebody* there that could help us out with a donation again this year?"

I couldn't believe what I was hearing!

"No, sir," I responded a little too firmly. "I'm afraid *no one* at *this* number can help you out."

He hung up on me.

Since then, I ask God for grace, sensitivity, and *wisdom* to know how to respond to others going through times of pain, especially if it's a type of pain I've never experienced myself.

In isolation with grief

Near midnight on the eve of Mother's memorial service, Darrell, who was working the night shift, came in to take my vital signs and check my IVs. Because I hadn't kept food down for three days, the doctor had added glucose to my IV menu.

Planning Mother's memorial service the previous week had given me a purpose to hang on. Psychologically, I'd put cancer on hold while traveling with Mother through her crisis. Now, for the first time since my diagnosis, I was alone with reality.

Too weak and nauseated to read or write, I began to suspect that life would go on . . . but I probably wouldn't.

"Looks like you're having a tough go of it," Darrell said quietly as he took the blood pressure cuff off my arm.

"Yeah" was all I could respond.

"I'll be back soon," he promised.

My physical pain was great that night, but it paled in comparison with the hurt of Mother's death.

Tears streamed down both sides of my bald head, reached the white cotton cap over my scalp, and were absorbed into its fabric.

I shivered under the blankets.

God? I silently ventured. *I guess You're about the only one anymore who doesn't need rubber gloves to touch me.*

I'm here in Room 2327, Bed A. I'm lonely and scared. Where are You?[2] *I really need to know, because I think it's boiled down to You and me. Tonight—You're all I've got.*

A still small voice spoke to my heart.

That's right. I am all you've got.[3]

Just Me—Jesus.

Jesus only

"Jesus only," as the apostle Matthew once put it. Recounting the story of Christ's transfiguration, he states that when Peter, James, and John opened their eyes after witnessing Christ's glorification on the mountain, they saw "Jesus only" (Matthew 17:8).

He "was in all points tempted like as we are, yet without sin."
—Hebrews 4:15

That night in the hospital Jesus was the only one that I could see, though I admit that I couldn't see Him very clearly.

The warmth from the invisible doorway leading toward death suggested that my life was slipping away.

God, I said, *I'm tired of holding on. Couldn't You maybe just let me die?*

A long soul silence ensued.

Then two unsolicited thoughts pushed into my clouded mind. The first was *But Carolyn, aren't you interested in knowing what I want regarding your future?*

The second thought was *A death wish doesn't usually come from My throne. Do you really want to play so easily into the hand of the enemy?*

I wondered, *Does this mean the final decision is up to me?*

Slowly my clouded mind began to suspect that two very important decisions would be made that night. One would take place in heaven. The other, in Bed A of Room 2327. Heaven would decide whether or not to keep me alive. My decision would be whether or not I'd accept God's will—even if it meant having to stay alive.

Tears flowing freely again, I suddenly recalled reading at one time that when we need it most, we can request our guardian angel to flash to heaven's throne for the purpose of bringing back reinforcement in the form of a second angel.[4] In my misery I didn't know if I really wanted to make that request.

But finally in a weak thought-prayer I prayed, *God, I'm at the end of my rope. If You will for me to die, hey, I'm up for that! Yet, if it's not Your will for me right now, please, could You send me a second angel to give me enough strength to show up for life tomorrow morning?*

I didn't see or hear or feel the arrival of that second angel to my hospital room that midnight hour. Yet into my thoughts came previously memorized words of comfort: "This I recall to my mind, therefore have I hope. It is of the Lord's mercies that we are not consumed, because his compassions fail not. They are new every morning: great is thy faithfulness" (Lamentations 3:21-23).

O God, I prayed. *I know You are compassionate, but do You really understand what I'm going through?*

As if in response to my question, I saw, in slow motion through the mists of my mind, a crude cross rising into the heavens and bearing the ultimate Sufferer. Then I knew. He understood.

As I clung to Jesus that night, He comforted me as only He could.

He's already been there

Through whatever dark valley *your* cancer is taking you right now—in terms of loss, pain, emotional anguish, or grief—He who hung on the cross in your place has already been there. Richard Stenbakken once said, "Wherever I go, He's been."[5]

You see, no one *understands* our pain better than Jesus does. He knows, from personal experience, just how desperately sin hurts. No one better than Jesus can truly *empathize* with the hurt it causes us (Isaiah 51:12).

Only the afflicted One can comfort the afflicted (Isaiah 53; 49:13).

Only Jesus, who lost loved ones Himself, can number the tears we shed (Psalm 27:10; 56:8; John 11:35).

The cruelest part of my emotional pain was the reality that no one—not my husband, not my son, nor my brother, nor my aunt— could get close enough physically to touch me. Likewise, on the cross Jesus was removed from those who would have physically comforted Him.

Perhaps that's why He promised to set up residence *within* His followers—and that includes you and me (John 14:21, 23)! That means He can actually draw closer to us than our very pain.

What a comforting thought! Yet that night I wondered: *Will He draw closer to strengthen me, or simply to hold me while I die?*

But before long I began to realize that maybe the answer to that question really didn't matter anymore.

Not long after midnight I made the choice to surrender my temporal life, my husband, my children, my relatives, my unspoken words, my unwritten books, my grief, my health, my destiny . . . *everything* . . . to Him.

Then I visualized my guardian angel on the left, standing beside the invisible artichoke bouquet. To the right, the recently arrived second angel—holding my hand through the guardrail—smiled over my shopping network list of prospective purchases.

And Jesus, who had somehow made this journey before me, stood at the head of my bed just beyond my pillow, bending over me . . . and making the final decision. In my mind's eye He came closer and gathered me to Himself.

Perhaps Darrell's checking of my vital signs would awaken me to the morning of my mother's memorial service. On the other hand, maybe I'd just go to sleep until the trumpet of God summoned me from my grave on resurrection day.

Either way, I now knew, would be just fine with me (Romans 14:8).

At last I drifted into a peaceful sleep, leaning fully—perhaps for the first time in my life—on the very heart of God.

REMINDER
We can lean on God's heart by knowing that Jesus, the ultimate sufferer, is closer to us than any pain we're experiencing (Hebrews 4:15).

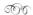

MEDITATION

A practical application of John 13:23 (personal paraphrase):
"One of Jesus' disciples, the one Jesus loved [you, or me perhaps?],
was leaning on God's heart."

---

[1] Interestingly enough, Al B. Weir, M.D., points out in his book *When Your Doctor Has Bad News* (Grand Rapids: Zondervan, 2003) that "a companion question to 'Why me?' is the question 'Now that I'm here, where are You, God?'" (p. 81).

[2] See Isaiah 45:21.

[3] Mike Mason, *The Gospel According to Job,* p. 84.

[4] See Ellen G. White, *Early Writings* (Washington, D.C.: Review and Herald Pub. Assn., 1882, 1945), p. 39; see also Hebrews 1:14 in the context of Revelation 5:11.

[5] At Cohutta Springs Conference Center, Cohutta Springs, Georgia, March 24, 2002.

Chapter 12

The Mirror of the Cross

"Lord, forget the cancer, only heal my soul."
—*My prayer, toward the end, based on Psalm 41:4*

The next morning a volunteer from the hospital chaplain's department stepped inside my room and scrubbed her hands. "Good morning," she said. "How are you doing?"

Just before she entered my room, I'd been thinking about my low white blood count. I'd also recalled how Proverbs 3:7, 8 states that fearing God and shunning evil "will bring health to your body" (NIV) and "marrow to thy bones" (KJV). So I tried to respond to her question by saying I was trying to "fear God" so my bone marrow would start producing more white blood cells. I'm afraid my mumbled response didn't make a whole lot of sense to her.

She took a few steps toward the window and then glanced from wall to wall. (For a minute I wondered if they had her on some of the same stuff they had me on!)

Then the woman approached my bedside. With a warm smile and taking care not to disturb the IV entry site, the volunteer took my right hand in hers and said, "I really don't know who you are. But do you know how refreshing it is to walk into a room in this oncology unit where there's a sense of hope in something beyond the grave?"

I looked up at her face.

She continued, "I can just *feel* God's presence in this room!"

I'd said nothing about hope in something beyond the grave. Her astounding words not only increased my sense of peace but also confirmed—as far as I was concerned—the presence of my second angel, whom I'd requested the previous midnight hour.

What comfort. What indescribable comfort during a time of personal pain and suffering!

The comfort of the cross

Regarding pain and suffering, Greg Boyd wrote in a letter to his unbelieving son: "For a great many this life is indeed filled with nothing more than pain and suffering, but from an eternal perspective, this is only a small part of the whole story. Jesus died on the cross so humans could exist eternally in the peace and joy of God—heaven—and the promise of Scripture is that this state of being will be such that our present sufferings can't be compared to it" (Romans 8:18).[1]

Each Christian in crisis—and crisis *will* come—must grapple with this most fundamental of questions: What will I do about the cross?

Will I continue to place my faith in the long-term promise of the cross for both this life and the hereafter, or will I give in to my current fears and give up?

The cross of Christ—and what it means both for my present and my future—is what finally brought peace to my heart during my journey through cancer. In fact, I would propose that the promise of the cross is the *only* reality that can bring temporal peace to a believer. Yet to those who don't understand this, how trivial the subject can become.

Just three days after my mother's death, I was surfing television channels in order to find something companionable in the background as I worked on her memorial service. The vivacious manner of an attractive saleswoman on a home shopping network caught my attention. She held several necklaces on a velvet-covered display board. The ornate pendants at the end of their gold chains were all in the shape of a cross.

With amazement I listened to her sales pitch: "Regardless of your faith, these pieces of jewelry are still very fashionable!"

Then the woman's cohost announced that a caller had just phoned in with a testimonial about one of these crosses she'd recently purchased from this shopping network. The cohost put the caller on the air.

To be perfectly honest, my mind leaped to the conclusion that the caller would tell how wearing her newly purchased cross had healed her of back pain or something similar. Instead the woman gushed, "The cross I bought from you ladies has absolutely changed my life! I used to be a yellow-gold person in terms of my wardrobe jewelry, but this cross has gotten me started wearing *white*-gold jewelry. This is an absolute transformation for me!"

Internal transformation, however, is what heaven intended should happen when you and I embrace the cross of Calvary—because of who hung there.

Perhaps those trivializing the cross do so because they haven't yet seen themselves in the *mirror* of the cross.

"Although the world is full of suffering, it is full also of the overcoming of it."

—Helen Keller [2]

Naked *on* the cross

During my bout with cancer I had frequently prayed that I'd come out on the other side a different person—whether I lived or died. God continues to answer that prayer in what I call the mirror of the cross.

To me Christ's physical nakedness on the cross is a spiritual representation that He had nothing to hide. When, during that dark night in ICU, I beheld in my mind's eye His transparency on the cross, it also reflected what I really looked like. I saw that it reflected my true self as clearly as a mirror reveals smudges on a dirty face.

Naked *before* the cross

Two out-of-state high school classmates, Milli and Judy, dropped by the hospital after Mom's memorial service. What a comfort they were! Then Rosie—a precious nonjudgmental friend who always helps me see life for what it is—came.

A subsequent journal entry records our conversation and what the mirror of the cross revealed to me.

April 20, 2003—*The evening of Mother's memorial service, my friend Rosie came to visit me. We talked about life and death and what that means in terms of who we really are.*

I told her that before cancer, I'd always wanted people to think I was strong. I controlled my emotions in public. I tried to smooth over how I was really feeling in order to protect the feelings of others. I downplayed the negative to the point of occasionally being dishonest about how I was really doing.

Why? I don't know. After all, even David—the man after God's own heart—captured his tearful laments in psalm after psalm.

I thought I could make really tough situations for people around me better. Again, I don't know why I thought this. Only Jesus can do that.

I realize I also wanted control over other people's opinions of me. Therefore, I was guarded in what I said about myself to them lest they judge me.

"Then the Lord said to Satan, 'Have you considered my servant Job? . . . He still maintains his integrity.' "

—Job 2:3, NIV

I told Rosie that my physical cancer had revealed a deeper spiritual cancer: pride, pride, and more pride.

She pointed out that pride in our lives often boils down to lies, lies, and more lies.

I shared with her that cancer had taught me to start living more transparently no matter what someone else might be thinking or saying. Rosie calls that living with integrity.

I told her that cancer had also taught me that I don't have to be a super mom or a super daughter or a super wife or a super friend—in short, Superwoman. Because in the end, I'm not! Trying to appear as such would just be another . . . lie.

God would much rather have me be an honest mom, an honest daughter, an honest wife, an honest friend—in short, an honest woman.

Jesus hung on the cross in a state of nakedness—a state of authenticity and transparency. The mirror of the cross showed me that, likewise, He wants me to live every moment of my life as authentically as He lived His.

Through the mirror of the cross the One who is acquainted with my grief and who has already experienced my pain (Isaiah 53) also brought my focus more directly on Him (Hebrews 12:1, 2), rather than on the me I was trying to protect . . . or cover up. . . or present as something I really wasn't.

Truly, my cancer has eaten to the core of a sinful heart. Perhaps that is the hidden blessing in this time of brokenness.

Commitment to authenticity

When I was eventually allowed to have visitors, I tried to be completely honest.

Without whining, I told them how badly I'd been hurting. (After all, Job told his friends *and* God!)

I told them how much I missed Mom and how grieved I was at not being able to attend her memorial service.

I told them that fear was a demon I encountered again and again.

I told them that I believed this was a testing time.

I also told them that I believed that God was still in charge and that I had found His throne to be more approachable than I'd ever imagined (Hebrews 4:16). What comfort—to both my body and my soul—God has given as I've worked purposefully toward authenticity, transparency, and total honesty.

More than ever I want Jesus to be my supreme example. In the Garden of Gethsemane and on the cross Jesus was honest about His suffering *and* His humanity (Matthew 26:38; John 19:28).

What a comfort, what a strength, to know that the One who intercedes for us has also experienced, with integrity, your cancer and mine—no matter what it is (Hebrews 4:15).

What a comfort His integrity can be to us. We can know with surety that He is not only the author of our faith (which grows stronger during the tough times in our lives), but also the finisher of our faith (Hebrews 12:2).

Indeed, G. Campbell Morgan wrote, "It is impossible . . . to see in Him man's wounded God, without becoming conscious of a great comfort and of a great strength."[3]

This strength includes the strength we need to live our lives with authenticity and transparency before the mirror of the cross—whether or not God chooses to deliver us from our cancers.

May the mirror of the cross reveal that our lives—by His grace—reflect the same strength and attitudes of the supreme Sufferer. The One who, when at the end of His rope, declared with perfect peace, "Father, into your hands I commit my spirit" (Luke 23:46, NIV).

REMINDER

We lean on God's heart by being completely honest with Him and with others about who we are and what we're suffering.

MEDITATION

"I lay down and slept; I awoke, for the
Lord sustained me" (Psalm 3:5, NKJV).

By the way, this verse is from one of King David's lament psalms. The more I journey through cancer, physical and otherwise, the more closely I embrace the psalms of lament. One Bible commentator has held up each of the lament psalms as "a model of godly response to suffering. The Lord does not expect us to remain stoic when we face suffering. We can pour out our souls to the Lord. However, in the middle of our cry we must remember God's loving care for us in the past so we can willingly trust Him with the future. With this type of response we can renew our hope in the living Lord."[4]

Some other lament psalms: 4-7, 12, 13, 16, 17, 22 (which also prophesies of Christ's future lament), 25, 26, 28, 31, 35, 38, and 41-44.

---

[1] Dr. Greg A. Boyd and Edward K. Boyd, *Letters From a Skeptic* (Colorado Springs, Colo.: Cook Communications Ministries, 1994), p. 27.

[2] In *Optimism* (1903).

[3] G. Campbell Morgan, *The Crises of the Christ* (New York: Fleming H. Revell Co., 1903), p. 404.

[4] "In Depth: The Psalms of Lament," *The Nelson Study Bible,* NKJV (Nashville: Thomas Nelson Publishers, 1997), p. 886.

Part III

Second Wind

*"Remember ye not the former things, neither consider the things of old.
Behold, I will do a new thing; now it shall spring forth; shall ye not know it?
I will even make a way in the wilderness, and rivers in the desert."*
—Isaiah 43:18, 19

I was only 9 years old. Yet I knew I was going to die.

After class one day, my fellow third grader, Sabrina, and I were giving each other free rides on our school's merry-go-round.

The ride I'd just given Sabrina ground to a halt, so she hopped off and start pushing the merry-go-round for me.

Soon her strong, stocky arms propelled the merry-go-round—and me—in delirious circles.

"I can make it go even faster!" she promised, energized by my squeals of delight. Once again Sabrina leaned forward, and, catching one of the gray metal bars with her hands, gave the spinning merry-go-round one final burst of speed.

On that rotation, however, I slammed into Sabrina's unwary elbow, my stomach taking the full brunt of the blow.

The next thing I remember was lying spread-eagled facedown upon the playground's rough asphalt. I could not breathe! When I tried to inhale, I felt as if my whole abdominal infrastructure had simply imploded.

I'm dying! I thought. *Mom and Daddy won't know what happened to me. I'll never see Wally or Pat [our dog] again!* I wanted to ask Sabrina to tell them goodbye for me, but I couldn't even draw a breath, much less talk.

105

LEANING ON GOD'S HEART

The terrified Sabrina hovered over my head, tearfully repeating, "Are you OK? Are you OK? What's the matter? I'm so sorry."

On my feet again

Then when I least expected it, I felt a tiny hint of fresh air quietly filter into my lungs. Then another. And another, and suddenly I realized that I could breathe again. I wasn't going to die after all!

I'd experienced what we adults sometimes refer to as a second wind.

In Part I we dealt with the topic of uncertain times. We explored eight ways that God provides for us in order to lean on His heart when a threatening personal storm—an unanticipated cancer—propels us into a time of uncertainty.

In Part II we looked at four ways by which God enables us to lean on His heart when a personal crisis forces us to the end of our rope.

Let's recap.

- We lean on God's heart by honestly grieving our losses before Him.
- We lean on God's heart when we allow compassionate people to support and comfort us.
- We lean on God's heart by acknowledging that Jesus, the ultimate sufferer, wants to be closer to us than any pain we might be suffering.
- We lean on God's heart in the midst of our crisis by being completely honest with Him and others about who we are.

In Part III we'll talk about godly responses to best-case scenarios, when God gives us a second wind and a reprieve from our pain. We'll also talk about godly responses to worst-case scenarios, those times God chooses not to heal our cancers.

Chapter 13

Learning to Trust More Deeply
(by Keepin' on the Sunny Side)

"Trust in the Lord with all thine heart;
and lean not unto thine own understanding.
In all thy ways acknowledge him, and he shall direct thy paths."
—Proverbs 3:5, 6

I settled into the daily hospital routine with the faint hope that perhaps God was indeed sparing my life—for the present, anyway. I resolved to do my part, as little as that might be, to make the best of this ordeal.

Though I couldn't yet read without becoming instantly nauseated, I asked God to help me at least recall previously memorized texts of comfort.

The word *victory* kept coming to mind. So did a flagship text of mine, John 16:33: "In the world ye shall have tribulation: but be of good cheer; I have overcome the world." I remembered that John also wrote that the victory that overcomes the world is our faith (1 John 5:4), our choice to *trust* in God.

I recalled a text memorized as a child: "Trust in the Lord with all thine heart; and lean not unto thine own understanding" (Proverbs 3:5).

In the privacy of my heart I asked God, *How can I better trust You in my situation?*

His answer to my heart was *Just praise Me for "our" victories.*

So I began to praise.

Yeah, God! Look how much water I've kept down without vomiting: two whole ounces. That's two more than the last time I tried.

107

Praise You, Lord! I didn't need help with my bath today. They let me sit up and do it myself. Hurray!

Wow! A whole spoonful of applesauce, and it's staying down! What a winner I am—with You here.

I made it all the way to the bathroom by myself. Way to go, Sutton! And thank You, God!

The dawn of a new day

As my white blood count continued to rise, my doctor permitted an occasional visitor. A girlfriend. A prayer partner. Then one wonderful day the doctor said my room was no longer in isolation.

Soon after she lifted the isolation ban Megan, a little girl from my own church congregation, came with her father to visit me. She was bearing a cheerful bouquet. She had come to the hospital that day for a spinal tap. In fact, she'd been in chemotherapy longer than I had—for leukemia.

Her beautiful little face (framed by a floppy hat, as she was also bald) gave me more hope and brought me more joy than she'll ever know.

As a measure of strength returned and as I kept down more food, the doctor let me go on short walks *outside* my room as long as I wore a mask over my nose. The first time I stepped out into the hall—the land of the living and the purposeful—I was as excited as if the queen herself had invited me to step into the entryway of Buckingham Palace!

Not long after, the doctor deemed it safe enough for me to share my room with another patient.

You're trusting Me through praise. Now trust Me to help you start serving others again, God instructed.

In here, *Lord? How?*

I'll let you know.

My new roommate, Greta (not her real name), was an elderly woman from the East Coast who had fallen while visiting her children there in Oregon. Extremely forgetful, she suddenly couldn't remember how to call the nurse.

"I need the nurse! I need the nurse!" Greta cried out that first afternoon.

"Just a minute, Greta," I said, pushing the call button on my bed. When the nursing station responded, I said, "The patient in Bed B needs a nurse."

"Oh, thank you," Greta sighed in relief.

Thank You, God, for giving me something to do for You right here in Bed A. I felt stronger already.

Looking ahead

Something else I did in the hospital to exercise my trust in God was to focus on the future. Before my cancer diagnosis I had previously agreed, along with some musician friends, to put on a Mother's Day program at a little church in the mountains north of Grants Pass. I'd also committed, before knowing I'd be hospitalized, to help put on a musical program at the assisted living residence where my mother had last lived.

This latter commitment was very close to my heart. Being back at "Mom's place" for the first time since her hospitalization and death would give me an opportunity to thank her friends for their support and prayers.

One of the musical numbers we'd planned to present for these events was "Keep on the Sunny Side of Life." Both Jim and my friends expressed doubt that I'd be well enough to participate in either function, yet I decided to trust that I'd be able to make these commitments. More than that, I practiced the music in my head, *mentally* skipping the little wooden hammers over the strings of my dulcimer.

Most of all, though I was still lying in a hospital bed, I rehearsed the words to this song even though I wasn't one of the vocalists. I especially liked the phrase in the chorus that proclaims that keeping on the sunny side of life will "help us every day and will brighten all our way."

Gladiola bulbs and pink roses

When I could finally have flowers in my room, friends sent

them. One friend sent an exquisite hand-painted ceramic pot holding a miniature rosebush. I chose those fresh, tiny blooms, not only as symbols of a new kind of trust in my life, but as symbols of the blessings in each of my *todays*.

Another friend gave me some very typically brown (and unattractive) gladiola bulbs. With the bulbs she included a pair of flowered garden gloves and a trowel. Her gift helped me focus on my *tomorrows*. For her handwritten card contained this message: "Dear Carolyn, spring isn't far off. My prayer is that when it arrives, you will be feeling well enough to plant these bulbs and enjoy God's blessing of renewal in your own life!"

"The gratitude which flows from our lips is the result of the Spirit's striking the cords of the soul in holy memories, awakening the music of the heart."

—Ellen G. White[2]

As the nausea subsided, I was able to start reading again. How the promises of Psalms and Isaiah and others encouraged me.[1] I picked up Scripture memorization where I'd left off, and found myself starting to think more clearly again.

Home again

One memorable morning, nine days after being rushed to the hospital and one week after Mother's memorial service, my doctor discharged me—with careful instructions concerning the many precautions I must now take. I didn't know how long I'd be out of the hospital. After all, Darrell had told me some cancer patients bounce in and out of the hospital like yo-yos. Some make it. Others don't.

I did know, however, that I could no longer trust *my* understanding of *anything*. So, leaning on my husband's arm—and leaning on the Overcomer of sin's cancer—I was able to clamber up the two steps from the garage into our house.

Home again. A week earlier this moment had seemed impossible.

Within an hour my fellow youth department leader arrived with a huge basket from our kids at church. Cards, stuffed animals, a lap throw, a neck pillow, self-portrait photos, a video of themselves singing hymns of encouragement for me, bubble bath, and cologne.

Discreetly tucked away in the bottom of the basket was a kit of hair products whose packaging promised to stimulate the scalp and encourage new hair growth. Bless their sweet hearts!

And yes, my hair *did* begin growing back in. First, a peach fuzz stage and then a silver satin that slowly spread over my scalp.

May 25, 2003—As my hair grows back in, I'm learning some things about my scalp. My hair grows in a circular motion, starting at the crown and continuing for the most part around my head. We're talking major cowlick here! No wonder I've always had trouble with my hair separating up there, no matter what style I'm wearing.

Also at the very front of my hairline is a two-inch-long-by-one-inch-deep cowlick. The ends of the cowlick grow in two opposite directions. So that's why my bangs have always wanted to go their separate ways! My hair is growing in thick, curly, and silver-gray.

At home I continued to celebrate small victories and take on new challenges. Since I'd lost so much weight, I decided to make myself four simple badly needed cotton skirts to wear during the hot summer months. Though I had almost no extra energy yet, I still made those skirts—one seam at a time. I took several weeks to complete this project, yet was surprised at how much I could accomplish when those little victories keep adding up.

Though I couldn't touch our cats because of the risk of contamination, I still enjoyed the companionship of Priscilla and Pansy Panther. I wasn't yet strong enough for long walks in the sun. Yet every day the cats and I took a single stroll around Jim's well-manicured garden.

Jim's major contribution to my sunny side of life was planting eight flower boxes on the back porch where I could see the spring blooms from the kitchen table. Soon a riot of floral hues, plus the babbling of a newly installed water fountain on the back deck, rejuvenated my weary soul.

Of course, I sometimes reached for the telephone to share with Mom my latest health progress or tell her how many hummingbirds were bathing in the fountain. Then I'd remember, and the tears would come. Frequently Jim would join me in a good cry.

Yet the sun continued to burst through spring showers. Robins'

111

songs sweetened the early-morning air. A volunteer tulip pushed up beside the little cottonwood in the front yard. Each new day was a gift just waiting to be opened and savored.

Some encouraging (musical) notes

And yes, I *did* make it to both of the musical performances for which I'd mentally practiced while still in the hospital. Two huge victories along my road to recovery.

As the others sang "Keep on the Sunny Side" at my mother's former residence, my little dulcimer hammers pounded out harmonic filler accompaniment. Never mind that I had to sit down between musical numbers or that my wig slipped a bit too far back on my forehead when I played. What was important at this point in my journey was focusing on the sunny side—and living there—through trust in God's being in control of my uncertain future.

An anonymous e-mail quote someone once sent me groused, "The trouble with life is there's no background music." I beg to differ. No matter how mundane or laborious or painful our days may be, we can always choose to hear the background music. Zephaniah 3:17 states that God "will rejoice over you with singing" (NIV). And let me tell you that is some serious background music!

Comfort from the throne

One day in early June I awoke from a disturbing dream. In my dream I'd been enjoying a good chat with Mother. Naturally, when I came to my senses, I remembered—yet again—that she was gone. Giving free rein to my emotions, I sobbed like a baby.

A bit later I wrote in my journal, *This is a testing day—a day to trust Him and cling to His promises. After all, "God withdrew from Hezekiah in order to test him and see what was really in his heart" (2 Chronicles 32:31, NLT).*

Dear God, I'm really missing my parents today. I don't even feel like eating—and we both know I need to put some weight back on. Please, Lord, comfort me. Today. Any way You choose. I need You!

Three hours later the telephone rang. A familiar, warm voice from my childhood said, "Carolyn, this is Aunt Arlene [my mother's maid of honor and longtime family friend]. I don't know why, but I have been thinking about you the past three days. Then right after lunch I had an overwhelming urge to phone. I guess I'm wondering if you need a mother today."

Wow! After that most welcome call I tearfully thanked God for comforting me in such a specific manner.

Around 4:00 that afternoon Jim brought home the mail and tossed what looked like a marketing letter of some sort into my lap. The return address identified the sender as the Review and Herald Publishing Association.

Assuming the envelope contained a bill (since I'd recently ordered some books from them), I unfolded the letter inside. The first word I saw was "Congratulations!"

What I next read nearly sent me into a state of ecstatic shock. This publishing company had accepted *Write It on Your Heart,* the manuscript on which Mother and I had collaborated just before her death!

I was about to tell Jim, who was still sorting through mail, when I noted I was holding not one sheet of paper but two.

In amazement I read the first paragraph of the second sheet of paper.

"While I live I will praise the Lord; I will sing praises to my God while I have my being."

—Psalm 146:2, NKJV

Now tears streamed down my face. The Review had also accepted the manuscript I'd finished between my surgery and first chemotherapy treatment.[3]

In response to my sniffles Jim looked up from a letter in his hand and asked with sudden concern in his voice, "What is it? Are you all right? What are you reading?"

"Oh, I'm fine," I sobbed. "Don't worry—I'm just being *comforted!* By God!"

Two facts about the acceptance of those book manuscripts still amaze me. First, the timing of the acceptance letters. They arrived within hours after I'd trusted God to comfort me that day. Second, I realized that had I not been facing cancer and Mother's decline, I probably never would have completed those writing projects in the first place.

Little by little I've been getting a handle on why the apostle Peter told us to rejoice in our trials (1 Peter 4:12, 13). It's through our trials that God's comfort, care, and glory shine the most brightly. God may not take away our storm clouds, but He certainly knows how to line them with silver. Those silver linings remind me to rejoice in "the sunny side"—the positive results—of my trials, even when I don't know what their outcome will be.

Christ focused on "the sunny side" as He hung on the cross in our behalf. He foresaw, through the eyes of faith, that His death would make possible your *eternal* salvation and mine (Hebrews 12:2).

Now, *that* is truly something to sing about!

REMINDER
We can lean on God's heart by keeping on the sunny side
through trust as we praise God for even small victories,
as we serve others, as we watch for today's blessings
and focus on tomorrow's promises.

MEDITATION
"He [Jesus on the cross] shall see the travail of his soul [you and me—His reason for dying], and shall be satisfied" (Isaiah 53:11).

---

[1] Promises to which I clung included Psalms 11:4; 45:6; 103:19; Hebrews 4:14-16; and Revelation 20:11.

[2] Ellen G. White manuscript 50, 1900.

[3] The two books were subsequently published as *Staying Vertical: A Spiritual Tool Kit for Christ-centered Living in an Out-of-balance World* and *Write It on Your Heart: How to Make Journaling Work for You.*

Chapter 14

When God Chooses Not to Heal

*"Do you want to hold out by clinging to your unfinished
life expectations and dreams, or do you want to hold on to Me?"*
—God, to me during my post-cancer journey

Just now I'm sitting before a picture window looking out over an azure, ripple-wrinkled lake here in north-central Michigan. Above the screen of the laptop perched on my knees I spot a pair of Canadian geese gliding past the lakefront prayer gazebo—just below my balcony.

I've been here in this pristine paradise for a week and a half, to speak at a women's retreat on three consecutive weekends. Day after day I've watched these two geese. In the morning they settle down on the sidewalk next to the gazebo. There they groom themselves as the sun rises over the evergreens and warms the cement beneath their feet.

Sometimes in the afternoon they mount the little hill outside my bathroom window and feed on insects. My two feathered acquaintances are used to me now in my red Camp Au Sable baseball cap and windbreaker as I start or finish my daily trek around the lake.

I wish them well, this magnificent pair of Canadian geese. I wish them well because last night I heard a pack of coyotes nearby. Their eerie yipping and howling sent chills down my spine.

I say a little prayer for the geese.

And I say a little prayer for me.

For as the echoing howl of preying coyotes carries long into the night, so does the lingering thought that my cancer might someday return to prey on me.

As a cancer survivor, I can never be considered a total cure—this side of heaven.

Of course, my treatment, both the medical and the natural, may have eradicated my cancer for good. I'd like to think that's the case. On the other hand, I may be a walking, breathing time bomb with undetected cancer cells preparing to explode inside my tissue when I least expect them to.

So, if you don't mind my doing so, I'm going to write this chapter for me. And, of course, for those of you who are grappling with how to respond when God does not heal our cancers. Someday I may need this chapter more than anything else I've ever written. I may need it to remind me of what's really important in this life and in the life to come.

I want to remember three things about my journey through any cancer. First, what cancer can do to me. Next, what cancer *cannot* do to me. And third, how God would have a child of His respond to terminal cancer of any kind.

What cancer can do to me

Yes, it can cause unspeakable destruction. Cancer can waste away my body. It can sap my strength and destroy my organs. It can stop me from traveling and publicly sharing God's goodness.

Cancer can stop me from experiencing life as I have been experiencing it, rich with variety and activity.

Cancer can break my husband's heart and leave my children motherless. Cancer can prevent me from watching my only grandchild mature into a beautiful young woman.

What cancer cannot do to me

On the other hand, cancer *cannot* change who I am. The woman whom God has been molding through life's darkest surprises and most amazing blessings.

Cancer *cannot* control my attitudes or my emotions. It may take my hair, but not my smile! Cancer *cannot* keep my spirit from dancing or my heart from singing (Psalm 30:11, 12).

116

Cancer *cannot* rob my loved ones of unforgettable memories of treasured family times.

And finally, cancer can *never* separate me from God!

A Christian response

How should a child of God respond to terminal cancer—whatever that cancer may be?

A spirit of surrender to God's sovereignty will always characterize a Christian's response. He or she will simply want to be at the spiritual, physical, and emotional place God has chosen for that day of life. David (Psalm 31:5), Jesus (Luke 23:46), and Stephen (Acts 7:59) all surrendered to heaven's will.

Job surrendered with the words "Though he slay me, yet will I trust in him" (Job 13:15). One writer has said that with these words of Job, God "won his wager with Satan."[1] If perchance God has entrusted me with cancer, then I want Him to win in my case as well.

If I eventually die from the disease, I want my final prayer requests to be these.

> "As with the cross, our darkest hour may be God's finest moment."
> —Mark M. Yarbrough[2]

- Let me breathe my last *believing God's unfulfilled promises,* knowing as did Abel, Abraham, and Sarah that I'll experience their complete fulfillment in heaven (Hebrews 11:13).
- Let me breathe my last *with a spirit of patience and gratitude.* John Newton's wife died of an illness that started as a huge tumor in her breast. Of his dying wife Newton wrote, "[God] gave her sweetness and patience. When I would say, 'You suffer greatly,' she would answer, 'I do suffer, but not greatly.' And she often expressed her thankfulness that, though she couldn't move her body, she was still able to use her hands."[3]
- Let me breathe my last *with my personal affairs in order.* May I have made everything right with both God and people. On the other side I don't want to learn that my real enemies weren't cancer cells, after all, but rather bitterness, anger, discouragement, or unfinished business.

- Let me die with *God's praise on my lips* and words of love and encouragement for those at my side. I can't help remembering my blind mother bidding us good night with these words: "I'm going to go to sleep tonight counting my blessings. I have so many."
- Let me breathe my last *with God's big picture clearly in mind.* Christ gave Peter, James, and John a glimpse of the big picture on the Mount of Transfiguration. Peter was so overwhelmed with Christ's glory that he exclaimed, "Lord, it is good for us to be here" (Matthew 17:4).

"If you think life is not fair . . . you're right!"
—Anonymous

However, when Peter descended the mount and encountered public chaos surrounding a self-destructive demon-possessed boy, he neglected to repeat the words "It is good for us to be here." Yet, why not? Peter was still with Jesus. May I daily draw close to Him because it is always good to be with Jesus—especially at the moment of death.

- Let me breathe my last *longing for home,* as I realize that I am but a pilgrim here (see Hebrews 11:13). Jesus clearly understood that He was but a pilgrim on this earth. Yet He "endured for the 'joy that was set before him' (Hebrews 12:2), and God's grace allows us to do the same," writes Mark Yarbrough. "Our affliction is purposeful and passing, and although we may not be able to understand it, we must cling to God's goodness."[4] After all, this world of pain, sin, and unfairness is not our home.

Chemo breakdown

Do you remember my sharing in an earlier chapter about a little song I wrote? I wrote it the morning I stood over the bathroom sink, gazing in the mirror with horror as unprovoked strands of my bangs did silent free falls into the sink. At that moment I realized that the chemotherapy side effect of hair loss had become a reality in my life.

Would you like to hear that little song I wrote through my tears and sang a few minutes later to my husband at the breakfast table? It's really a song about longing for home. Being in a bluegrass mood that day, I entitled my homely composition "The Chemo Breakdown." However, its spiritual title is "This World Is Definitely *Not* My Home!"

The Chemo Breakdown

Hair falling out by handfuls, I'm as weak as I can be.
    Feel like a total stranger on this chemotherapy.
But I'll just keep a smile—can't keep a good woman down
    When her sights are set on heaven . . . and a golden crown.

Chorus:
In the end, in the end.
    I know where I'm going in the end.
Awaiting up in heaven is my great Physician-Friend,
    So I know where I'm going in the end.

Well, I'm a sitting duck for every bug that comes around.
    It's hard to beat the odds when your immunity is down,
Wearing wigs and old bandannas—yet my Lord won't let me down—
    For a balding head looks glorious . . . 'neath a golden crown.

Chorus:
In the end, in the end.
    I know where I'm going in the end.
At the end of every rope, I'll choose to cling to heaven's hope,
    For I know where I'm going in the end.

Yes, I'm going up to heaven, and it's very clear to me
    Ain't no clinics up in heaven with first floor oncology.
So if He takes me now, or if He takes me then . . .
    I still know where I'm going in the end.

Chorus:
In the end, in the end.
 I know where I'm going in the end.
So I'll just do my part by leaning on His loving heart,
 For I know where I'm going in the end.
© 2006 by Carolyn Sutton

David Biebel writes that "while we hurt from the pain of it all, and we long for the freedom of the glory of the children of God, we can also see by faith where everything is heading. Our comfort and hope is knowing that He will one day make it right again."[5]

Final thoughts beside the lake

As I watch this pair of Canadian geese glide around the grassy point and out of sight, I review what I have written this afternoon. Lord willing, I won't need to reread this chapter . . . if God prevents a return of the cancer.

"But if not," as Shadrach, Meshach, and Abednego would say, then I would add one final request of God. That request is this.

Let me breathe my last *leaning on the heart of the One who loves me best.* The heart of the Pearl of great price, whose exquisite beauty was formed through a lifetime of intense suffering. For "I want to know Christ and the power of his resurrection and the fellowship of sharing in his sufferings, becoming like him in his death, and so, somehow, to attain to the resurrection from the dead" (Philippians 3:10, 11, NIV).

With my last breath, let me tell my precious Lord, "As for me, I will behold thy face in righteousness: I shall be satisfied, when I awake, with thy likeness" (Psalm 17:15).

For in the end—as my little song humbly points out—"no one living in Zion will say, 'I am ill' " (Isaiah 33:24, NIV).

REMINDER

Even when God chooses not to heal our cancers, we can still lean on His heart by realizing that neither cancer nor anything else can ever separate us from God or from the power of His resurrection.

120

⌒⊙⌒

MEDITATION

"Behold, I tell you a mystery: We shall not all sleep, but we shall all be changed—in a moment, in the twinkling of an eye, at the last trumpet. . . . The dead will be raised incorruptible. . . . And this mortal must put on immortality. . . . 'Death is swallowed up in victory'"
(1 Corinthians 15:51-54, NKJV).
"Therefore comfort one another with these words"
(1 Thessalonians 4:18, NKJV).

---

[1] Mike Mason, *The Gospel According to Job,* p. 153.
[2] Mark M. Yarbrough, "When God Doesn't Heal."
[3] *John Newton, Letters of a Slave Trader Freed by God's Grace,* par. Dick Bohrer, p. 114.
[4] Yarbrough.
[5] David Biebel, *If God Is So Good, Why Do I Hurt So Bad?* p. 134.

Chapter 15

On the Road Again—
And Traveling Light!

"Success is not final, failure is not fatal;
it is the courage to continue that counts."
—Winston Churchill

From horizontal to vertical.

From stationary to mobile, and on the road again!

No, God's enabling of these positive changes in my life didn't occur overnight. They came gradually. Day by day. Month by month, with generous doses of fresh air, water, rest, sunshine, homemade fruit and veggie juices, increasing daily exercise, and continual praise to the trustworthy One that I was still alive.

Some areas of my renewed life, though, had a different perspective now.

Although I was pushing 59, I had just become an official orphan. That took some getting used to, both mentally and emotionally.

Being down and out for several weeks had also impacted my psyche.

After nearly three months of being quasi-dependent, I found it difficult to get up the nerve to drive again. Before my illness, I'd been a fairly assertive driver. Now I realized how deadly cancer can be to one's self-esteem. After a few short trips to the grocery store, however, my road confidence returned. Soon I felt as if I'd never stopped driving.

As my immune system showed increasing signs of a comeback, my doctor gave me permission to travel by air without having to be quite so fearful of contracting other people's airborne illnesses.

I thought back to Bed A, in Room 2327. On my back and totally dependent on others, I'd not dared think that, even if I lived, I'd ever be strong enough to serve God in any significant manner.

While I was still wearing a wig, Corleen Johnson, who had providentially phoned me just after Mother's death, called to ask if I felt up to presenting a single seminar at a one-day convocation in central Oregon. Inwardly I questioned my being equal to the task. After praying about her request for a couple of days, I agreed. After all, the only way to assess my abilities was to make a stab at using them. During the presentation a few weeks later I was surprised at how strong I felt.

Five months later a women's ministries leader—this time in central Oregon—phoned to say that her speaker had had to cancel for her upcoming two-day retreat.

Would I be able to fill in the following weekend, just three days from then?

She also mentioned, as an aside, that she was looking for a preacher to fill the pulpit of a nearby church, as her preacher-husband (who also served as a chaplain with the National Guard) had just been called to Iraq. Again, after praying about her requests, Jim and I accepted.

Since then, to our own amazement, we have spent much of our time on the road.

A travel dilemma

One aspect about traveling I've always dreaded is the prejourney decision-making about what goes into my suitcase for any given trip. Invariably I take either too many warm clothes or not enough hot-weather garments. Perhaps the size of my suitcase necessitates leaving behind an extra pair of shoes in favor of tennies for walking.

Recently, however, I attended a seminar concerning Christian dress. The lovely presenter included ideas on how to pack a clothing capsule for a trip. She showed us (wide-eyed!) participants how to select and pack just six key clothing items that could be expanded into—believe it or not—45 different outfits!

Since attending that seminar, I've been traveling a whole lot lighter than I used to.

Traveling lighter . . . through life

Likewise, since cancer, I've also been traveling a whole lot lighter.

Gone is excess baggage I used to haul around with me . . . needless worry . . . fear . . . regret . . . disappointment. Cancer has helped me understand what's most important to take with me for the rest of my spiritual journey.

As with the capsule suitcase wardrobe, I've narrowed down my spiritual travel wardrobe to a basic six. Six God-given essentials that I can mix and match.

Would you like to peek inside my suitcase?

Suitcase essential 1: hope

In my travels I've found the garment that best flatters and enhances the other five is *hope*. Hope is my anchor, both "sure and stedfast" (Hebrews 6:19). Hope is the key to keeping my heart strong (Psalm 31:24). Hope will see me through to the end of my journey (1 Peter 1:3, 13).

"Suffering changes us, but worry drains us."
—Donald Hilliard, Jr.[1]

Not by coincidence did the psalmists end their writings with renewed calls for hope in God (Psalms 42:11; 43:5). As Christian "cancer" survivors, our hope is both in God (Psalm 130:7; Lamentations 3:24) and in the truth and promises of His Word (Psalm 130:5).

Why is hope so essential in our spiritual wardrobes? Because, in the words of cancer survivor Dr. Amy Givler, "hope looks ahead."[2]

Concerning hope as it relates to cancer, Dr. Givler states, "Cancer is conquerable. People who are hopeful handle the bumpy road ahead better and are happier with the life they are living as they are going through treatment. It doesn't have to be a hope for cure, or even for remission. Hoping for freedom from pain, for growth as a person, and for quality time with family members may be just as satisfying as hoping to live to reach 90."[3]

Hope expects Him who began a good work in us to complete it

(Philippians 1:6). Through the sacrifice of Christ we have a hope that goes beyond suffering (Hebrews 5:8, 9). Hope assures us that God will make all things right in the end (1 Peter 1:13).

Suitcase essential 2: joy

The second essential garment in my spiritual travel wardrobe capsule is *joy*. Joylessness, on the other hand, leads to depression, and depression hampers healing.[4] Proverbs 17:22 reminds us that "a merry heart doeth good like a medicine." That's why I designated one section of my pre-cancer treatment notebook for lighthearted sayings and quotations.

However, I didn't realize the practical health benefits of a good hearty laugh until I ran across the following information.

"Dr. William Fry, Jr., of the Department of Psychiatry at Stanford Medical School, likens laughter to a form of physical exercise. It causes huffing and puffing, speeds up the heart rate, raises blood pressure, accelerates breathing, increases oxygen consumption, gives the muscles of the face and stomach a workout, and relaxes muscles not involved in laughing. Twenty seconds of laughter, he has contended, can double the heart rate for three to five minutes. That is the equivalent of three minutes of strenuous rowing."[5]

"In the sentence of life, the devil may be a comma—but never let him be the period."

—Unknown

How important it is for us to practice joy! When I returned home from the hospital and starting receiving visitors, two close girlfriends came to visit me. They had also been wonderful support to my mother up until the very end.

In addition to "The Chemo Breakdown," I had written another song during my cancer journey about other medical issues. I started to sing the song for them. Suddenly something struck them so funny that they simply slumped over in their chairs, doubled over with laughter. The sight of their being so out of control gave Jim and me the giggles. Soon the four of us were holding our sides, wiping our eyes, gasping for breath, and reaching for the tissue box.

I like to imagine that God was in the center of this merry gathering, helping us unload some of our grief and sadness through a good belly laugh. After all, David said of God, "Surely you have . . . made him glad with the joy of your presence" (Psalm 21:6, NIV). I suspect a whole lot of healing took place that afternoon, for all of us.

Have *you* had a good wholesome laugh recently—for your *health's* sake?

By the way, one of the best methods of enhancing our sense of joy is to be openly grateful to God for the unmerited favor He constantly showers upon us. An unknown writer once stated that he who forgets the language of gratitude can never be on speaking terms with joy.[6]

How true!

Suitcase essential 3: courage

The third essential garment in my spiritual suitcase is *courage*.

American poet Maya Angelou has written, "Without courage, we cannot practice any other virtue with consistency. We can't be kind, true, merciful, generous, or honest."[7]

One of the attributes I most admire about the apostle Paul was his dauntless courage. After recounting the trials he'd suffered at the hands of his enemies—and the certain danger in his immediate future—Paul made this astounding statement: "But none of these things move me; nor do I count my life dear to myself, so that I may finish my race with joy, and the ministry which I received from the Lord Jesus, to testify to the gospel of the grace of God" (Acts 20:24, NKJV).

Because of his courage, Paul persevered when the going got tough.

Author Mike Mason observes that "not all Christians, in short, are going to be blessed with healthy bodies, well-balanced characters, or obviously fruitful ministries. . . . Such believers may not be conquerors, but they are 'more than conquerors' (Romans 8:37)—that is, they are something better than conquerors, since they hold to their faith in the midst of apparent defeat."[8]

Paul courageously held on to his faith. Of him author Ellen White writes, "His lips had been touched with a live coal from off the altar, and he was enabled to rise above *bodily infirmities* and to present Jesus as the sinner's only hope."[9]

Another writer notes, "Most of the world's useful work is done by people who are pressed for time, or are tired, or don't feel well."[10] They simply persevere—compelled by *courage* to keep going.

Lord, especially in this day and age, give us courage!

Suitcase essential 4: purpose

The fourth essential garment in my spiritual travel wardrobe capsule is a sense of *purpose*.

Two and a half months after losing Mother and being unexpectedly hospitalized myself, I refined and rewrote my personal mission statement. Precisely *because* of my painful journey through cancer, I now have a more biblically based purpose than I did before. You might say that since cancer, I take the Bible, not necessarily more literally, but more personally.

"The joy of the Lord is your strength."

—Nehemiah 8:10

I find my mandate in John 4:34. It is to do God's will for my life and help finish His work here on earth.

Do you know *your* purpose at this stage of your journey? God will help you identify what it is. And when you recognize your God-ordained mission, He will empower you to go to work with a passion you've never before experienced.

Beware, however. God will also *stretch* you. He certainly has me.

One other thing: God doesn't want us to be content with just smoldering beneath the radar. He wants us to be on fire.

In a Northern state I recently visited in a home that was heated by a wood-burning stove. Evidently something was wrong with the flue, for the house had filled up with smoke. I couldn't help but thinking about God's aversion to a lukewarm state of soul (Revelation 3:15, 16). He'd probably agree with a rustic sign I bought my husband to hang in his workshop: "If yer smokin', you'd better be on fire!"

A strong sense of purpose sharpens us mentally, brightens our emotional outlook, and puts pep in our step. It energizes us.

Suitcase essential 5: caring people

The fifth essential garment in my spiritual travel wardrobe is *caring people*.

Again, Dr. Givler notes, "A number of studies show that signs of better immune system function increase as people have more emotional support and tangible social support. Friendships and close family relationships buffer people from the negative effects of stress."[11]

I thank God for the family members and friends who buffered me during my time of overwhelming stress. A card here, a phone call there. Perfectly timed e-mails with just the right Bible encouragements. A Federal Expressed flower bulb to water and then watch as it grew into a towering golden amaryllis.

Having come so close, during my medical crisis, to losing these treasured people for good, I consider them gifts from God. Their gestures of compassion and concern make me want to do the same for others who need buffering.

Suitcase essential 6: love

The sixth essential garment in my spiritual travel wardrobe capsule is *love*. His love for me.

I owe Him everything. After all, I shouldn't still be here today.

Sometimes people who conjecture about my experience say, "Well, God must have spared your life because He had something more for you to do."

That may be true.

However, I suspect the greater truth is that God spared my life because He had something to do . . . *in* . . . me. And I am most grateful for His love-powered patience.

That's why these days, when invited to share Him and what He's done for me, I just go. I go for *Him*. Whether on the road . . . in the air . . . or facing a television camera (*way* out of my comfort zone), I'm there! I'm there—because He loves me.

Bottom line?

I've shed the excess baggage.

I'm free at last.

My journey through cancer—and through anything—can't ever be about me again. It will always be about Him. Because Jesus is enough.

And He's the reason I'm traveling a whole lot lighter these days.

REMINDER

We lean on God's heart by traveling life's road with just the essentials: hope, joy, courage, purpose, caring people, and God's overarching, eternal love.

MEDITATION

"I have discarded everything else, counting it all as garbage, so that I may have Christ. . . . As a result, I can really know Christ. . . . I can learn what it means to suffer with him, . . . so that, somehow, I can experience the resurrection from the dead"
(Philippians 3:8-11, NLT).

---

[1] Donald Hilliard, Jr., *Faith in the Face of Fear* (Mobile, Ala.: Evergreen Press, 2002), p. 75.

[2] Amy Givler, *Hope in the Face of Cancer,* p. 29.

[3] *Ibid.,* p. 27.

[4] *Ibid.,* p. 168.

[5] Norman Cousins, *Head First, the Biology of Hope* (New York: E. P. Dutton, 1989), p. 132.

[6] Vern McLellan, comp., *The Complete Book of Practical Proverbs and Wacky Wit* (Wheaton, Ill.: Tyndale House Publishers, Inc., 1996), p. 222.

[7] In the Dayton, Tennessee, *Herald-News,* Apr. 17, 2005, p. A-6.

[8] Mike Mason, *The Gospel According to Job,* p. 260.

[9] Ellen G. White, *The Acts of the Apostles* (Mountain View, Calif.: Pacific Press Pub. Assn., 1911), p. 208. (Italics supplied.)

[10] In McLellan, p. 247.

[11] Givler, p. 171.

EPILOGUE

Are We at Bethsaida Yet?

"Uncertainty is here to stay.
Situations may resolve. Relationships may heal.
But uncertainty in a sinful world won't end until Jesus comes.
Learn to live with it!"
—A lesson cancer taught me

While embarking on a little Horizon Air jet not long ago, I noticed a heading posted on the inside wall above the emergency exit row. It simply stated, "Suitability Criteria of Exit-Seat Occupants." Then it listed the requirements of those who might need to remove the emergency doors to help other passengers escape during an in-flight emergency.

I think back to the biblical storm story we discussed in the introduction to Part I of this book. You'll remember that, after feeding the 5,000, Christ instructed His disciples to go across the Sea of Galilee toward Bethsaida. Then an unexpected storm arose, blowing the disciples' boat off course.

Just when the disciples needed Jesus most, He appeared to them walking across the raging sea. He called. They responded. They were in contact. Yet the fury of the storm did not automatically abate just because they were praying (which is what talking to Jesus is).

Likewise, just because we pray in the midst of a personal crisis doesn't mean the storm—or in our case, the cancer—will *automatically* go away.

I like to think of the disciples on that stormy night as exit-seat occupants traveling in that little boat being tossed by vicious waves. Christ had chosen them to help others escape from the power of sin. Soon He would commission them to take the gospel to the world.

Yet they needed a bit more training and experience themselves before they could meet the criteria for exit-seat occupants. So Jesus let the storm continue to rage.

You may recall that the most impulsive exit-seat occupant, Peter, actually *exited* the boat. He asked Jesus if he could also walk on the troubled waters. Christ granted his request, calling Peter to His side. Then Peter, despite the storm raging about him, walked atop the waves—as long as he kept his eyes on Jesus.

A special promise

Just before His crucifixion Jesus made a special promise to those who loved Him. He promised (in John 14:21) to reveal Himself to all those who lean on His heart by submitting everything about their cancers to Him. Of course, that's *my* paraphrase of the principle in that text (within the context of this book). Nevertheless, that promise is for modern-day exit-seat occupants—you and me—as much as it was for the original 12 disciples.

I don't know how God is going to reveal Himself to you in your situation, but I'll tell you about a time He revealed Himself to me.

I was going through a cancer journey—the cancer of divorce—when God quietly manifested Himself to me *beside* the Pacific Ocean (rather than walking *on* it). He did so through an itinerant writer who was trying to make a few quick bucks on the boardwalk of California's colorful Venice Beach.

That particular summer afternoon I took my troubled heart on a stroll along the boardwalk. I remember trying to make sense of recent events in my life and wondering how to pick up the pieces.

I made my way between the oceanside stalls of vendors hawking their wares. A Rollerblading man wearing a turban and flowing white robes nearly skated into me. That's because he was trying to avoid hitting the crowd gathered around the sword-swallowers. (You get the picture.)

I found myself behind a group of people standing before a little man sitting on a straight-backed chair. He pounded away on an old-fashioned typewriter that stood on a collapsible table.

This man was a smaller version of Superman's alter ego, Clark Kent. White dress-shirt sleeves rolled up to his elbows, horn-rimmed glasses, necktie loosely knotted, the brim of his Depression-style journalist hat pulled over one eye, a press card stuck in the hatband.

A sign beside the typewriter boldly introduced him as "The world-renown 60-second novelist. Your autobiography for only $5."

Fascinated, I watched the man finish and hand a typed page to a woman in front of me while graciously emphasizing, "The story of your life, ma'am."

She paid him.

I thought, *Boy, he sure saw* her *coming—and fleeced her big-time!*

Then, with a small hourglass in his hand, the 60-second novelist was suddenly looking up at me. "Miss," he said in a professional yet friendly manner, "may I write for you—in the next minute—a deeply relevant novel based on the story of your life? Only $5."

I laughed in spite of myself and then grew sober. Life wasn't funny anymore.

"God promises a safe landing, not a calm passage." *

—Unknown

Feeling safe behind anonymity, I blurted out, "First of all, I'm not a Miss *or* a Mrs. In fact, I don't *what* I am anymore!" Recent shock and grief expelled more unexpected words from my lips. "My marriage just blew apart. I never expected to be divorced! I don't think I even have a life anymore. So there's *nothing* to write about, really. I'm just here visiting relatives who live on a boat." (And to think my father had always told me from an early age, "Don't tell the neighbors *everything* you know!")

The man expertly lined up a sheet of paper and rolled it into the carriage of his little typewriter.

"My dear," he said with a winsome smile, "there's *always* something to write about. What's your first name, please?"

"Carolyn," I responded involuntarily, unwarily walking into his marketing trap.

"Carolyn," he said, "I want to thank you for giving me the makings of a blockbuster novel." With that he turned over the little hourglass on his table and pounded away at the typewriter keys.

The last grains of sand slipped into the base of the hourglass just as the 60-second novelist proficiently ripped the paper from the typewriter, spinning its carriage in the process. He neatly folded the page in half, revealing a precopied cover on the reverse side.

"Here you go, Carolyn," he said with a broad smile, holding out the "novel" to me with both hands. "It's bound to be a best seller."

"Yeah, right," I said, rolling my eyes and reaching into my handbag for the $5 out of which I'd just been hoodwinked.

Down at the beach a few minutes later, I sat on a bench and drew from my bag the 60-second novel. The bare-bones account of a hero named Carolyn.

"Carolyn once felt she was on the firm rock of a solid marriage. Yes, she was married for 22 years. Then it crashed on the rocks.

"Carolyn sent out an SOS, but it was too late . . . she knew not what to do. But she dived into the water, the rough waves of chance and opportunity. And she swam to the shore of stability again. Now it's been a year, and she's even been visiting her brother's boat, where he lives moored to the dock."

(Had I told him all that?)

"And Carolyn realized that she never really had been on land—that we're always on the water ready to jump overboard at a moment's notice. So she hasn't gotten her land legs back yet, although she's feeling pretty good. Because she just might not be a landlubber after all."

A special promise . . . fulfilled

Through the novelist's words "the rough waves of chance and opportunity" God gave me an unlikely reminder that He is the author of second chances and the Creator of new opportunities.

After all, He's told us in Isaiah 43:18, 19, "Do not remember the former things, nor consider the things of old. Behold, I will do a *new* thing" (NKJV).

I once heard a TV lecturer state that the Chinese character for the word *crisis* has two possible definitions: one is "danger"; the other is "opportunity."

Though it was a long shot, I suddenly wondered if the 60-second novelist might not be on to something. He'd also written about me, "She just might not be a landlubber after all." Maybe—according to the principle of Romans 8:28, where God says He can make all things work together for our good—just maybe God had something else for me to do still. Obviously it would no longer be on the solid footing of a longtime marriage, yet perhaps I'd find it in the uncertain waters of my new singlehood.

Maybe I *was* a swimmer and just didn't know it!

And you?

What about *you*? Where are you in your cancer storm? Holding on to the sides of the boat as a contrary wind blows you off course on your way to Bethsaida? Perhaps an exit-seat occupant wondering if it's time yet to exit? The question "Why?" may continue to demand an answer. Or else you're wondering, *What's the purpose of my storm right now?*

Well, friend, if I didn't receive any concrete "Because . . ." answers in *my* storm, I certainly don't have any for you. However, let's consider several possibilities.

First, our storms may have to do with our growing stronger *spiritual* muscles as we hold on for dear life, simultaneously surrendering heart, mind, and soul to the Master of the wind and waves.

Then again, our storms may involve our being thrown into the sea . . . only to be rescued and washed by the blood of the Lamb as He prepares us for something new in our lives—to use the word that Isaiah did (Isaiah 43:19; see also 1 Peter 1:7; Job 23:10).

Finally, our storms may be about uncertainty and waiting, about *treading water—in His strength*—as we await guidance from the still small voice amid the howling winds.

Christ, the same today

Above the roar of our clamoring Why, we hear the voice of the Master speaking to us. What Emmanuel said to His disciples in the

135

Galilean boat that midnight hour, He also says to you and me at this very moment: "Be of good cheer. I am with you."

"Fear not, for I have redeemed you; I have summoned you by name; you are mine. When you pass through the waters, I will be with you; and when you pass through the rivers, they will not sweep over you. . . . For I am the Lord, your God. . . . Since you are precious and honored in my sight, and because I love you" (Isaiah 43:1-4, NIV).

Remember that impetuous exit-seat occupant, Peter? Christ was with him when he walked through the waves. Do you know what happens to us exit-seat occupants as well when, throwing caution to the wind, we run across the waves of our storms to Jesus? The Author of second chances and the Creator of new opportunities transforms us from mere survivors into overcomers. He shapes us into energizing examples of how to live—and die—with eternal hope in His love.

Rather than desperately struggling to reach Bethsaida (or numerous other locations, such as Finding the Perfect Husband, or State of Perfect Health, or Perfect Financial Security), we courageously press forward, through our cancers—and *beyond*—to a place called Perfect Faith. This faith has been perfected by surviving—against the heart of God—any cancer that the devil or anything this dying world catapults our direction in terms of temptation, heartache, pain, or loss.

Peter's cancer was impetuosity, arrogance, and pride.

And Peter was drowning. Yet when he turned his eyes up on Jesus, he actually *walked* on water.

You know, of course, that God hasn't changed since that long-ago midnight storm. The same consistency and faithfulness that He manifested in Peter's life, He will without doubt manifest in yours and mine.

And when we, like Peter, keep our eyes upon Jesus *only* . . . our hand in His . . . our very soul leaning hard against His loving heart— He will enable us to walk on water through the cancers of trouble and trial, and—praise God—far, *far* beyond!

REMINDER

We lean on God's heart when we put our hand in Christ's,
despite life's cancer storms, and let Him lead us into a
no-matter-what faith that will sustain us until the end.

❦

MEDITATION

"I will cry to You, when my heart is overwhelmed;
lead me to the rock
that is higher than I" (Psalm 61:2, NKJV).

★ In Vern McLellan, comp., *The Complete Book of Practical Proverbs and Wacky Wit,* p. 8.

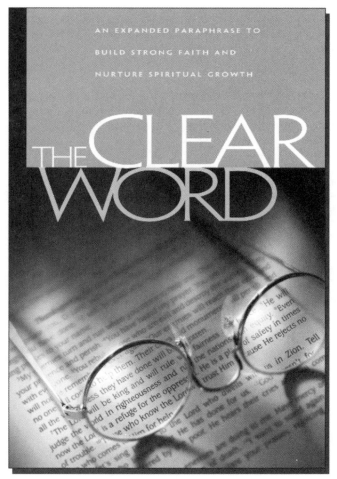

DISCOVER A LOVE THAT WILL CHANGE YOUR LIFE

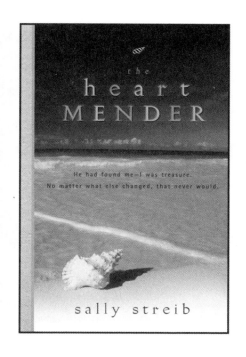

As a child and as a wife, Sally Streib was told that she was worthless, that she would never amount to anything. But her life journey proves how wrong humans can be. Now Sally shares her story of struggle and renewal—along with the biblical stories of other women restored by Jesus—and reveals how God's love can fill empty hearts with a sense of worth, purpose, and joy. 0-8280-1890-1. Paperback, 160 pages.

3 WAYS TO SHOP

- Visit your local ABC
- Call 1-800-765-6955
- www.AdventistBookCenter.com

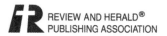